The London Lock Hospital in the Nineteenth Century

THE
London Lock Hospital
in the Nineteenth Century

GENDER, SEXUALITY AND SOCIAL REFORM

Maria Isabel Romero Ruiz

PETER LANG

Oxford·Bern·Berlin·Bruxelles·Frankfurt am Main·New York·Wien

Bibliographic information published by Die Deutsche Nationalbibliothek
Die Deutsche Nationalbibliothek lists this publication in the Deutsche
Nationalbibliografie; detailed bibliographic data is available on the
Internet at http://dnb.d-nb.de.

A catalogue record for this book is available from the British Library.

Library of Congress Control Number: 2014936829

Cover image: Plate showing the Lock Hospital in the nineteenth century.
Engraving by W. Walker from drawing by Thos. B. Sheperd, uncatalogued,
the Library, Royal College of Surgeons of England.

ISBN 978-3-0343-1727-6

© Peter Lang AG, International Academic Publishers, Bern 2014
Hochfeldstrasse 32, CH-3012 Bern, Switzerland
info@peterlang.com, www.peterlang.com, www.peterlang.net

All rights reserved.
All parts of this publication are protected by copyright.
Any utilisation outside the strict limits of the copyright law, without
the permission of the publisher, is forbidden and liable to prosecution.
This applies in particular to reproductions, translations, microfilming,
and storage and processing in electronic retrieval systems.

This publication has been peer reviewed.

*To my daughter Ana and my son Pepe,
my most precious treasure.*

Contents

List of Illustrations   ix

Acknowledgements   xi

CHAPTER 1
Introduction: The London Lock Hospital and Asylum
and Specialist Hospitals in the Nineteenth Century   1

CHAPTER 2
Fallen Women, Prostitutes and the Treatment
of Venereal Disease in the Nineteenth Century   25

CHAPTER 3
Female Patients and the Lock Hospital Regulations
throughout the Nineteenth Century   57

CHAPTER 4
The London Lock Hospital and the Contagious
Diseases Acts: Reports and Accounts   81

CHAPTER 5
From Deviancy to Purity: The London Lock
Asylum and Moral Reform   125

CHAPTER 6
The London Lock at the Turn of the Century:
New Perspectives on the Physical and
Moral Cure of Deviant Women   159

Bibliography   201

Index   211

Illustrations

Picture of Anne Sewell, 4th September 1850, Portrait by J. Holt, Patients' Records, the Library, Royal College of Surgeons of England, MS0022/6/6.   42

Picture of William Bentley, 23rd April 1850, Portrait by J. Holt, Patients' Records, the Library, Royal College of Surgeons of England, MS0022/6/6.   43

Picture of the child of Mary Ann Agnes, 2nd May 1850, Portrait by J. Holt, Patients' Records, the Library, Royal College of Surgeons of England, MS0022/6/6.   47

Front Cover Appeal for 6,000 pounds to complete the Asylum for Female Penitents, Cuttings Album, the Library, Royal College of Surgeons of England, MS0022/11.   77

Front Cover Report 1839, Cuttings Album, the Library, Royal College of Surgeons of England, MS0022/11.   131

Acknowledgements

This monograph is the result of many years of hard work on the issue of fallen women and prostitution in the nineteenth century in England and on the archives of the London Lock Hospital and Asylum which are kept in the Library of the Royal College of Surgeons of England, in Lincoln's Inn Fields, London.

My deepest gratitude goes first to my dear friend and colleague, Professor Logie Barrow from Bremen University, Germany, who is an academic with a solid career and academic prestige in the history of the working classes and the history of medicine in the United Kingdom. Without his support and advice this monograph would have never seen the light. I also want to express my gratitude to the librarians and archivists at the Library of the Royal College of Surgeons of England because they have always been helpful and supportive in the difficult process of taking notes from archival materials and locating manuscripts for my research. My special thanks go as well to my research leader and friend, Professor Pilar Cuder, and my colleague and friend, Dr. Beatriz Domínguez, both from the University of Huelva in Spain, for their constant encouragement and for believing in me as an academic; also, I wish to show my gratitude to my dear colleague, Dr. Blanca Krauel, from the University of Málaga, for being my friend and counselor through hard times of professional and personal challenges. I am also indebted to Professor Cora Kaplan from Queen Mary University of London, and Dr. Paulina Palmer, retired from Warwick University, who have always encouraged me in my academic projects and given me their friendship and advice. Finally, I would like to put in words my gratitude to my family, and especially to my parents and my children, who are my inspiration in life. To all of them I dedicate this work.

CHAPTER I

Introduction: The London Lock Hospital and Asylum and Specialist Hospitals in the Nineteenth Century

Although several publications have focused partially or as a whole on the London Lock Hospital and Asylum archives, which can be found at the Library, Royal College of Surgeons of England in London, none of them has taken into consideration the role of these two institutions in the rescue and cure of fallen women in the nineteenth century.

David Innes Williams in his 1995 book, *The London Lock: A Charitable Hospital, 1746–1952*, writes a careful history of the Hospital from its foundation in 1746 to its closure in 1952, analysing different periods in relation to aspects such as the treatment of venereal disease, medical theory and practice, the patients, the staff, the governors, finance, the Chapel and chaplains, the buildings and the situation of the Hospital and Asylum at the different stages of their existence. Williams' work constitutes a comprehensive volume essential for the scholar who wishes to have a general encompassing approach to the history of the hospital. A narrower aim is achieved in the case of the book published by Kevin Siena in 2004 entitled *Venereal Disease, Hospitals and the Urban Poor: London's Foul Wards 1600–1800*, which devotes two chapters to the London Lock. Throughout his work, Siena analyses the role of Royal Hospitals and Poor Law Infirmaries in the cure of venereal disease in the destitute poor as well as the creation of lock hospitals which came to complete the offer of medical institutions for "foul" patients in London. However, his endeavours to come to terms with the social and hospital treatment of the *pox* are centred on the history of the eighteenth century. The same happens with two other contributions that deal with the institution: Donna Andrew's chapter on the London Lock Hospital and the Lying-in Charity for Married Women included in the 1994 book by Jonathan Barry and Colin Jones *Medicine and Charity before the Welfare State*; and Linda Merions' 1997 edition *The Secret Malady: Venereal Disease in Eighteenth Century Britain and France*, where she writes a chapter where she explores the Lock Asylum for Women in the eighteenth century.

Other scholars have also focused their attention on different reform institutions and hospitals in the nineteenth century. One of them is Judith Walkowitz's *Prostitution and Victorian Society: Women, Class and the State* (1980), which touches on the Royal Albert and the Royal Portsmouth, which had lock wards for women in Southampton and Portsmouth respectively; another is Frances Finnegan, whose *Poverty and Prostitution: A Study of Victorian Prostitutes in York* (1979) talks about rescue and reform at the York Penitentiary. This Penitentiary had many similarities with the London Lock regarding the running of the institution, its propaganda to obtain funding and its aims at reforming and teaching prostitutes and fallen women; her later *Do Penance or Perish: A Study of Magdalene Asylums in Ireland* (2001) analyses the characteristics of these places of confinement in Ireland which were dominated by the Catholic approach to rescue work; and Linda Mahood's *The Magdalenes: Prostitution in the Nineteenth Century* (1990) deals with the Glasgow Lock Hospital and Asylum in several chapters as a an example of a Scottish institution for the reform and cure of Victorian prostitutes.

The topic of Victorian social reform on the part of the middle class and of private and public institutions for the cure and restitution of deviant women can also be found in the work of other scholars in a more general way. This is the case of social history writers such as Louise A. Jackson, focusing on social reform with fallen girls in her 2000 *Child Sexual Abuse in Victorian England*, and Paula Bartley, who writes about reform institutions in general, dealing with fallen women in *Prostitution: Prevention and Reform in England, 1860–1914*, also published in 2000.

This book aims throughout its chapters to analyse the London Lock Hospital and Asylum archives for the study of aspects concerning the cure of venereal disease in the nineteenth century and the treatment and reform of fallen women. Issues of gender and female sexuality will become the centre of debate together with the policing and regulation of deviancy

Introduction: The London Lock Hospital and Asylum

in the working classes, and particularly in women. For that, a brief history of the reform movement and the spread of specialist hospitals in England together with a history of the Hospital and Asylum will be included in order to establish the background for the treatment of venereal disease as far as prostitutes and fallen women are concerned. Similarly, the application of middle-class standards of behaviour and respectability will be studied in the light of Hospital regulations in the nineteenth century, and also in the functioning of the Asylum as an institution with the purpose of reforming female penitents and restoring them back to society as decent working-class women. After that, the impact of the application of the Contagious Diseases Acts in the running of this charity following the Reports and Accounts of those years will be the object of my concern. After that, focus will shift to the impact of the application of the Contagious Diseases Acts in the running of this charity via the Reports and Accounts around the time of those Acts. Finally, the changes brought about by the end of the century with their emphasis on child prostitution, white slavery and new perspectives on rescue work and purity, and the extension of the work of the Lock to other elements in the charity movement will round off my efforts to portray a critical image of the moral and medical activities carried out in the Hospital and Asylum to help those individuals suffering from extreme poverty and from the "most dreadful disease".

Specialist hospitals and voluntary hospitals began to proliferate in the eighteenth century. At the same time, modern medicine was born – at least if we follow what Foucault describes as "the birth of the clinic" with its associated expert ("clinical") gaze – and helped generate the new concept of hospital medicine.[1]

The case of British specialisation was especially slow and difficult in comparison with France and the rest of the continent, because it faced strong hostility. In the eighteenth century, there were bonesetters, dentists, oculists and specialists in venereal disease who were considered as quacks and worked outside the regular profession which was dominated

---

1   Kevin Siena, *Venereal Disease Hospitals and the Urban Poor: London's Foul Wards 1600–1800* (Rochester, New York: University of Rochester Press, 2004), 127.

by physicians and surgeons. Similarly, in the late eighteenth and early nineteenth centuries, specialist surgeons began to appear, becoming ophthalmic surgeons, surgeon-dentists and orthopaedic surgeons; however, the most popular field of specialisation was midwifery.[2]

The British medical profession was first divided into three groups: physicians, surgeons and apothecaries. The 1815 Apothecaries Act stipulated that licenciates of the Society of Apothecaries attend various lectures and pass its examinations; they also had to spend six months in a hospital, dispensary or infirmary to finish their training. At the beginning, surgeons had a lower social status than physicians and were allowed to treat patients externally but not internally; physicians thus constituted the elite of medical practice. Getting the education and training to become a doctor was very expensive, and medical men usually came from the upper classes. Scottish Universities like Edinburgh, Glasgow, St. Andrews and Aberdeen all had medical schools, so the majority of doctors graduated from them. At the beginning of the nineteenth century, most medical teaching was obtained from private schools and only three London Hospitals had medical schools: St. Bartholomew's, the United Hospitals (St. Thomas's and Guy's) and the London; similarly, the early 19th century saw the founding in London of two university colleges, King's and University, where medical teaching was carried on. But doctors also needed the training in hospitals to get qualified, and those who got their teaching from provincial medical schools in hospitals could sit this university's examinations. Oxford and Cambridge students could get their training and research in the London hospitals, but then they were examined by their universities.[3]

The passing of the 1858 Medical Act represented a crucial step in the history of British medicine. The old system of qualification by apprenticeship was substituted by a formal education based on lectures and written

---

2   George Weisz, "The Emergence of Medical Specialization in the Nineteenth Century", *Bulletin of the History of Medicine* 77, 3 (2003): 565.

3   Michelle Higgs, *Life in the Victorian Hospital* (Stroud, Gloucestershire: The History Press, 2009), 112–114. At this stage, medical students could obtain degrees of M.B. (Bachelor of Medicine) or Ch.B (Bachelor of Surgery), C.M. (Master of Surgery) and M.D. (Doctor of Medicine).

examinations based on a syllabus together with training in hospital wards and textbooks which would allow medical students to have a knowledge of a range of diseases in order to be able to identify and to treat them. This new legislation did not exclude certain "unqualified practitioners such as homeopaths, herbalists, naturopaths and quacks" but established the Medical Register which was published annually to ensure that all doctors were properly qualified. There were several medical corporations in Britain which included the Royal College of Physicians, the Royal College of Surgeons, the Society of Apothecaries and the Royal Colleges or Faculties in Edinburgh, Glasgow, and Dublin. Both these corporations and universities or hospital medical schools could now examine and certify candidates to practice medicine. With the Act, requirements and qualifications from medical schools were established and a General Medical Council was created to keep the Medical Register and to monitor the ethical and professional behaviour of doctors. Posts for which qualified doctors could apply were those in hospital consultancies, public vaccination, asylums, prisons, the colonies, the Poor Law and the public health service.[4]

The three categories of doctors were later replaced by General Practitioners and elite Consultants in the second half of the nineteenth century, and this fragmentation was certainly a serious obstacle in the process of specialisation of British medicine. The medical elite in the Royal Colleges saw the latter as a threat. This medical class did not want to lose their situation of power and privilege and, as a consequence, did not want to spread medical and clinical knowledge which was circumscribed to a circle of gentlemanly doctors who were appointed through a system of patronage to purchase hospital posts. The lack of a unified education system with competing hospitals and medical schools was equally a hindrance in the advancement of medical specialisation.[5]

Despite all this, an increasing number of specialist hospitals did appear in the eighteenth century, and this tendency continued growing in the

---

4   Ibid., 114–115.
5   Weisz, "The Emergence of Medical Specialization in the Nineteenth Century", 561–563.

nineteenth. These hospitals were usually private and catered for those patients who were not accepted in voluntary hospitals, like the mentally deranged, women in labour and those suffering from various types of fever and venereal disease. They were run with the support of philanthropists who could bring them a reputation and a rich private clientele. Many of these hospitals charged a certain amount of money for their services and became very popular among the middle classes as "they were 'free from the stigma of charity' which blighted general voluntary hospitals".[6] In the first half of the nineteenth century there were in London 27 specialist hospitals, infirmaries and dispensaries, of which 12 had survived from the eighteenth century, and 22 in the provinces. The Royal Colleges of Physicians and Surgeons did not want to accept specialist doctors among their members and such doctors were largely ignored in the medical press.[7] As a result, specialisation was taken up by ambitious doctors who had been excluded "for religious, educational or social reasons from posts in general hospitals",[8] establishing competing small institutions based on the philanthropic and voluntary model, representing a menace to the general voluntary hospitals as the public responded enthusiastically to this new endeavour. Examples of specialist hospitals established in the nineteenth century were the Eye and Ear Infirmary, later known as "Moorfields" opened in 1805, the Royal Ear Hospital run in Soho from 1816, St. Mark's Hospital for Fistula and other Rectal Diseases founded in 1835, the Royal Orthopaedic Hospital and the Metropolitan Ear and Throat Hospital both opened in 1838, the Brompton Hospital for lung and heart diseases founded in 1841, the Hospital for Sick Children established in 1850, and the National Hospital for Nervous Diseases set up in 1859.[9] Thus the natural consequence was that general hospitals began to add specialised departments to their traditional resources between 1855 and 1875, although they systematically appointed

---

6   Higgs, *Life in the Victorian Hospital*, 18.
7   Weisz, "The Emergence of Medical Specialization in the Nineteenth Century", 565–567.
8   Ibid., 566.
9   David Innes Williams, *The London Lock: A Charitable Hospital for Venereal Disease, 1746–1952* (London and New York: Royal Society of Medicine Press Ltd., 1995), 77.

Introduction: *The London Lock Hospital and Asylum* 7

non-specialists to their specific wards, but later in the century it began to be possible to develop a good specialist career in general hospitals. The reasons for the acceptance of this new situation were that Britain had to come to terms with European medicine which was based on clinical research and specialisation; the gradual intervention of the state in the health system; and the attempts at administrative and professional unity made by the advocates of medical reform.[10]

At the beginning of the eighteenth century, there were two major hospitals in London, St. Bartholomew's and St. Thomas's which had been founded by religious orders and were then taken over by the City of London, becoming Royal Hospitals. These hospitals had to admit any patient that required medical assistance, and they used to have "foul" wards or out-houses where the venereally diseased were treated. This period saw the birth of the Voluntary Hospital Movement which endorsed a health system for the poor that relied on charity.[11] Hospitals always had difficulty meeting their running costs as far as medical supplies, wages and maintenance of the buildings were concerned. Funding was obtained through a variety of sources which included voluntary subscriptions, church collections, bequests from wills and donations from benefactors, besides diverse charity events like annual fairs, musical festivals, sermons in the chapel, banquets, etc. Annual subscriptions were paid by rich or otherwise conspicuous members of the community, and this pecuniary contribution entitled them to become governors and recommend a certain number of in- or out-patients to the hospital per annum. Subscribers who paid an important sum could become governors for life. In this respect, the roles of the Treasurer and Collector were essential for keeping and increasing the number of annual subscriptions, and with that aim the role of the institutions in the cure and treatment of patients was praised in the propaganda found in Annual Accounts and the local press of the time.[12] Patients were to be treated

10 Weisz, "The Emergence of Medical Specialization in the Nineteenth Century", 568, 572–573.
11 Innes Williams, *The London Lock: A Charitable Hospital for Venereal Disease, 1746–1952*, 8–9.
12 Higgs, *Life in the Victorian Hospital*, 11–13.

free, and Physicians and Surgeons gave their services without receiving any salary; however, working for these charities gave them prestige and status in the community for the good effects of their generosity on these charitable concerns.[13] As we shall see, the London Lock Hospital was both a specialist and a voluntary hospital.

All these changes led to a radical transformation in the concept of illness which was based on the new corporeal paradigm born out of the new medical practice and concept of learning. Consequently, the old theory of humours was replaced by the vision of disease as physical lesions located in different parts of the body. Before that, illnesses were believed to be caused by the imbalance of humours or fluids which were the constituents of the body: black bile, yellow bile, phlegm, and blood; therefore, treatments were aimed at controlling the humoral imbalances, and popular ways of getting rid of "bad humours" were "bloodletting, sweating, vomiting, salivating, urinating and purging".[14] So, according to Siena, "Hospitals, where doctors and medical students performed an increasing number of dissections and saw an increasing number of cases, provided the forum for the birth of this new medicine".[15] This meant that the image of the body was more "objective" and the approach to medicine was more statistical and anonymous. Another important change is that the relationship between patient and doctor was transformed, and patients lost agency in the process as their symptoms were not the result of individual and intrinsic imbalance of humours but of uniform bodies that functioned in an identical but identifiable way.

As a result, hospital medicine became one more discourse of power and knowledge which created the category of the subject, together with other prisonlike institutions such as prisons, asylums, penitentiaries, workhouses, etc. These modern institutions were given the purpose of producing docile bodies through discipline and surveillance. In Foucauldian terms, "the carceral" makes inmates of these institutions behave according to norms,

---

13 Innes Williams, *The London Lock: A Charitable Hospital for Venereal Disease*, 9.
14 Higgs, *Life in the Victorian Hospital*, 71.
15 Siena, *Venereal Disease Hospitals and the Urban Poor: London's Foul Wards 1600–1800*, 127.

subordinates individuals to institutional needs, scrutinises and observes all subjects, and uses punishment to control deviants.[16] Thus power is not exercised by the state but by social institutions which create these "docile bodies". This idea, together with the fact that "modern power operates through continual classification, surveillance and intervention", ease the ascription of bodies to different categories (race, gender, illness, class, etc.) and different actions to rules that can be regarded as "praiseworthy, deviant, punishable, or criminal", as Foucault's volume I of *The History of Sexuality* establishes.[17] Following this reasoning, "foul patients" were deviant subjects who had not conformed to the rules of society as far as sexual performance was concerned, so their behaviour was punishable. In the case of women, sexual promiscuity was seen as an even more despicable fault than in men. In fact, their illness was the physical punishment for their sexual sins, and hospitals simultaneously provided them with the cure and controlled and contained them. Nonetheless, acts of insubordination were not uncommon, as will be later discussed.

The roots of the reform movement can be found in the seventeenth and eighteenth centuries, although most initiatives had a traditional halo, like the Societies for Reformation of Manners, which fought against the Biblical sins, that is, "vice, Sabbath-breaking and swearing", but they were mainly concerned with the ordinary people aspiring to have the lives of their social superiors. Christian reform took another direction when the Society for the Promotion of Christian Knowledge (SPCK) was founded in 1698. This Society focused on gin as the main cause of immorality among the poor and images of the fall of the Roman Empire were prevalent as an example of the consequences of vice. By the middle of the eighteenth century, reformers began to believe in social change through progress, and founded institutions like the Foundling Hospital (1741) for children, the Lock Hospital (1746) and the Magdalene Hospital (1758) for prostitutes.

---

16   Michel Foucault, *Discipline and Punish: The Birth of a Prison*, trans. Alan Sheridan (London: Penguin Books, 1979), 293–308.
17   Vincent B. Leitch, ed., *The Norton Anthology of Theory and Criticism* (New York and London: W-W-W Norton and Company, 2001), 1472.

These institutions' spirit was based on compassion rather than fear and loathe for "the undeserving" poor.[18] In the late eighteenth century and the early nineteenth, the traditional Puritanism of the middle classes was imposed on the aristocracy and the ungovernable poor, and Christian values were spread by people like the Wesleyan Methodists, the Benthamites and especially the Anglican Evangelicals, particularly the members of the Clapham Sect. These established the Proclamation Society in 1787 and the Society for the Suppression of Vice in 1802; they tried to close brothels and punish sexual offenders in the low orders, though morality was partially imposed on the aristocracy.[19]

Throughout the nineteenth century, several institutions ranging from penitentiaries and asylums to specialised homes were founded by middle-class philanthropists to rescue and reform prostitutes. Significantly, similar institutions were not created for men who had had recourse to prostitution as an escape for their sexual needs, following the Victorian assumption that men's sexual needs are stronger than those of women. Penitentiaries were the hallmark of both the Established Church of England and the Roman Catholic Church. In the middle of the century, the number of penitentiaries increased with the formation of the Church Penitentiary Association (CPA) inspired, unlike its imitators by the "High-Church" Oxford Movement. All this was due to an evangelical revival, which advocated an alternative system of rescue work based on a family system instead of a penitential one.[20] Paula Bartley argues that the name *home* for these institutions had connotations of domesticity, being woman's natural environment, but also of comfort and support.[21] However, the implications behind these institutions were even stronger: women were made dependent and submissive, and male and middle-class power was exercised over them. Asylums were run by members of the

---

18   Patrick Dillon, "The Roots of Reform", *History Today* 57, 3 (2003): 45–46.
19   Innes Williams, *The London Lock: A Charitable Hospital for Venereal Disease, 1746–1952*, 49–50.
20   Paula Bartley, *Prostitution: Prevention and Reform in England, 1860–1914* (London and New York: Routledge, 2000), 25–26.
21   Ibid., 30.

Church and also by lay men and women. The administrative and financial parts of these organisations were in the power of men, who also did the jobs connected with the public sphere such as attending meetings and courts, writing annual reports and publicising their work to get funding; women were in charge of the internal affairs, purchasing the goods and articles needed, supervising diets, dress and leisure of the inmates as well as their work to contribute to the running of the institution. Charity work was thus constructed around the lines of the gender division of labour which prevailed in other fields of human activity.

Before giving an account of the history of the London Lock Hospital and Asylum in the nineteenth century, we need to briefly analyse the history of institutions such as hospitals and workhouse infirmaries which were previously created or coexisted with the London Lock. It is important to have a clear appreciation of the presence and pre-eminence of venereal disease in all social classes in the eighteenth century, but its devastating nature was especially prevalent among the urban poor, and Londoners were continuously surrounded by the effects of this most-dreaded illness. There were two hospitals with venereal wards and outhouses for the destitute: St. Bartholomew's and St. Thomas's. Outhouses were initially built outside hospitals to keep lepers away from any contact with other patients or their families, but were later used to keep venereally diseased patients. The spirit behind them was always the same: leprosy had been the symbol of pestilence and degradation and that role was now played by the "foul disease". The idea was thus to avoid contact between venereal patients and "clean" patients, and for that purpose doors were locked and windows shut. Also the word *lock* had an implication of a social evil which was perceived as a peril in respectable society. It was used in former times to refer to hospitals where lepers were kept. Leprosy was then considered a very dangerous malady that had to be contained, and lepers were segregated from the rest of society to avoid the spread of this disease which provoked social panic. The people with means to pay privately for a doctor and treatment would never resort to either of these places. Both were Royal Hospitals financed by rents, not by donations, but charged an admission fee which, together with the public process of admission, had a punitive character. Patients were also segregated as the foul were separated from the clean in these hospitals, probably to avoid both moral and physical contagion.[22] It seems that there were more male patients than female; they were not required to have a nomination to obtain a bed, but a governor's intervention made things easier. Consistently with the then gendering of morality, women were usually considered as less worthy objects of charity than men by governors who, of course, were all male. However, people who stood as sureties were even more important in speeding admission to the hospital: this meant that someone had to post a bond for a patient to be treated.[23] Most bonds were posted by men, but there were also women who did this, and gender played a role here too: men preferred other men to pay bonds for them and women relied on other women. There was a whole business going on for people to get money for the bonds from victuallers or hospital staff who had their money returned with interest. From the mid-18th century, patients had also to put up with being observed and examined by medical students as part of the price of being cured of venereal disease, as these two hospitals were committed to treating those patients other institutions refused.[24]

Apart from the Royal Hospitals, Poor Law Infirmaries were the places where the poor could find relief. In the eighteenth century, workhouses worked under the Elizabethan Poor Law of 1601. Paupers had to have a settlement from the parish where they had been born that entitled them to poor relief, but there were other ways to obtain settlements through marriage, work or apprenticeship. Parish relief was supported from the rates that wealthier members of the community paid, and thanks to the efforts of the SPCK mentioned above, the 1723 Workhouse Test Act was passed. However, the initial idea of workhouses as places where work, profit and moral reform were furthered, gradually mutated into something different because of the health needs of their inmates, and workhouse infirmaries

---

22   Siena, *Venereal Disease Hospitals and the Urban Poor: London's Foul Wards 1600–1800*, 104–106.
23   The bond consisted in the payment of one guinea to cover the costs of burial, were the patient to die.
24   Siena, *Venereal Disease Hospitals and the Urban Poor: London's Foul Wards 1600–1800*, 111–119, 125.

Introduction: The London Lock Hospital and Asylum

developed. A physician or a surgeon and apothecary had to be contracted, but in most cases physicians did not earn a salary. Instead, their private practice would benefit from the experience of treating the poor, and they also gained prestige for their charity work within the local community.[25] Before the reforms of the 1860s, workhouse infirmaries were superintended by the matron and the master of the workhouse. There was also a paid nurse, but local women had to be employed as nurses usually recruited locally, as was the midwife. There were usually wards for men, for women, a lying-in ward and a ward for the mentally ill. Conditions were mostly as dreadful as in workhouses generally. The "foul" wards for people with venereal disease and other infections were in even worse condition than the others and segregation of men and women was applied.[26] The medical charitable network consisted of workhouse infirmaries as well as of royal hospitals and small specialist hospitals supported by voluntary subscription, and all these elements worked in collaboration to provide destitute people with medical treatment for "the pox". In fact, parishes paid for the hospital admission fees for their paupers, so the process of "passing" a pauper was not uncommon;[27] the salivation treatment lasted for about four to six weeks, and after that, "foul" patients sometimes had to be sent back to recover in the workhouse infirmary, before being released. The majority of workhouse inmates were women, old people and children who could find themselves in a much more desperate position than men. In the case of the salivation wards, the proportion of women was considerably higher, and most of them were in their early twenties and single.[28] This bears a correlation with the kind of female patients that were admitted into the London Lock Hospital, as we shall see. Premarital sex was quite common among the poor classes and in rural areas; in the eighteenth century, both

---

25 ibid., 136–139.
26 Higgs, *Life in the Victorian Hospital*, 28–30.
27 The fact of "passing a pauper" consisted in the process by which those paupers who did not have a settlement in the parish were returned to their own parish, after a huge amount of paperwork.
28 Siena, *Venereal Disease Hospitals and the Urban Poor: London's Foul Wards 1600–1800*, 161–166.

pregnancy outside marriage and venereal disease were a symbol of moral and sexual transgression. However, the expense incurred by a bastard child for a parish was so high that church wardens were especially stringent in the case of single mothers, although they viewed the pox as the result of sexual promiscuity. The character of the infected person was under scrutiny, except for the cases of wet-nurses who got the illness from an infected child, or decent wives, who had been infected by their immoral husbands. Workhouse discipline and rules were strictly enforced and this constituted a common feature of all charitable institutions during the period.

The London Lock Hospital was established by William Bromfield in 1746 for the cure of venereal disease, following the trend of voluntary and specialist hospitals in the eighteenth century. With the purpose of obtaining funding to open the Hospital, Bromfield advertised a meeting in St. Martin's Library to create the charity in two London newspapers, the *London Evening Post* and the *Daily Advertiser*, and interested parties would put the money for subscriptions through Drummond's Bank at Charing Cross. He managed to obtain the sum of 350 pounds to acquire the lease of the plot of land in Grosvenor Place, near Hyde Park Corner, and two wards with thirty beds, one for male patients and another one for female, were provided.[29]

William Bromfield (1712–1792) was a surgeon who came from a London family with a long medical tradition. At the beginning he was not very well-known, but in 1742 he became a Governor to St. George's Hospital, one of the Great Hospitals in London, which excluded venereal patients, and was elected Assistant Surgeon to the hospital in 1744, thus starting a prosperous and rewarding career. In 1745 he was appointed Surgeon to Frederick Prince of Wales, who was then President of St. George's Hospital; in 1769 he became Surgeon to the Queen's Household. Besides obtaining the money for the Lock Hospital, he contributed to the institution, participating in the Committee business and "recruiting Governors from amongst the aristocracy and from those in the theatrical

---

29 *A Short History of the London Lock Hospital and Rescue Home, 1746–1906* (The Library, Royal College of Surgeons of England, London), 3–4.

Introduction: The London Lock Hospital and Asylum 15

profession".[30] At the end of his professional life he had some medical and diagnostic disputes with other medical authorities like John Hunter and financial disputes with some of the Governors at the Lock, so it can be presumed that his last years were sad, especially after the deaths of most members of his family.

Although, traditionally, the London Lock Hospital has been seen as an institution for the cure and reform of moral sinners, following the spirit of moral improvement campaigns carried out by members of the Society for the Promotion of Christian Knowledge and the Society for the Reformation of Manners mentioned before, Siena argues that this was not the primary aim behind the foundation of the Lock during the first three decades of its existence. The change in attitude came about from the 1780s with the arrival of the Evangelicals who took control of the London Lock.[31] At this stage, there was a close relationship between the Lock Hospital and St. George's, which would continue till the end of the century, as many donors contributed to both institutions which shared medical staff and exchanged patients, so that the Lock became a kind of outhouse for St. George's Hospital. In these early days, there was an agreement with the Magdalene Charity and with the Foundling Hospital, which "paid for a special ward and nurse to attend the children sent by them".[32] However, in the Annual Reports of the nineteenth century children are hardly mentioned as patients in the Hospital.

The London Lock Hospital had the administrative structure of a voluntary hospital. There were annual subscriptions for those who paid five guineas and became governors for one year, and donors who paid fifty guineas became life governors. Governors could attend all meetings and vote, and sit on committees, like the board committee which met every Thursday to discuss hospital matters and the admittance of patients. Each governor could also recommend one patient at a time, and there were lesser

---

30   Innes Williams, *The London Lock: A Charitable Hospital for Venereal Disease, 1746–1952*, 11–15.
31   Siena, *Venereal Disease Hospitals and the Urban Poor: London's Foul Wards 1600–1800*, 182.
32   *A Short History of the London Lock Hospital and Rescue Home, 1746–1906*, 8.

donations without voting rights like those of many apothecaries; legacies were also very welcome. The list of Governors was published in the Annual Reports and Accounts and, at this early stage, it was stated that there was a number of lady subscribers whose names did not appear. During the first years the Hospital could meet hardly half of the expenses, so subscriptions had to be supplemented with a series of charitable events to raise funds such as concerts, plays, dinners and breakfasts. After all these efforts, the Charity was out of debt in 1753 and a third storey was added to the first building in 1766 "giving it the appearance familiar from the 19th-century print", after a fresh appeal had been made at a public meeting in St. James's Coffee House.[33] Initially, two physicians were appointed, Dr. Peter Shaw and Dr. Charles Cotes, who was replaced by Dr. Richard Conyers after his death two years later. These physicians left the, for them, lowlier routine of patient-care to the surgeons, who were credited for the treatment of nasty illnesses like those of venereal patients. The appointed surgeons were Bromfield himself and his assistant Dr. Thomas Williams, and there were several apothecaries. Similarly, a Divine was recruited as Chaplain to the Lock for visiting the patients in the wards. The early rules established that male and female patients could not mix and re-admissions were forbidden.[34]

Early Reports formulate the Hospital's focus as being on those among the poor who were suffering from venereal disease. To them would be added innocent wives and children, also prostitutes, so as to minimise the spread of contagion. The fact that there were no other institutions to which these kinds of infected patients could resort is also emphasised.[35] These arguments can be found again in the Annual Reports through the 1820s and 1830s, and the need for an institution of this sort could be read both in these and in the Accounts. For example, in that for 1837, we can read:

> The malady, to the cure of which the Lock Hospital is appropriated, peculiarly requires medical assistance; and if neglected, or improperly treated, it must terminate

---

[33] Innes Williams, *The London Lock: A Charitable Hospital for Venereal Disease, 1746–1952*, 24.
[34] Ibid., *1746–1952*, 22–23.
[35] Ibid., *1746–1952*, 21.

Introduction: The London Lock Hospital and Asylum

fatally by the most dreadful progress of lingering suffering; while, at the same time, it is more generable cured than most other diseases. We may indeed consider the dire distemper itself, as a declaration how greatly and holy God abhors licentiousness; yet hath he [sic] mercifully provided medicines which seldom fail, when judiciously used, to eradicate it completely. We ought, therefore, doubtless to imitate his [sic] compassion to the persons of the guilty, as well as the hatred of their crimes.[36]

Arguments of both God's abhorrence of the existence of promiscuity and of venereal disease and of God's mercy and compassion for these sinners were used to justify the need for the existence of the Institution. The idea that this was the only place where the most destitute infected with the pox could go to find medical assistance was put forward in the following words:

> When the Lock Hospital was founded, persons labouring under the dreadful disease were excluded from most of the Public Charities; they are still inadmissible into many Hospitals both in town and country: and though others have seen it necessary to make some provision for them, yet the *deposit* required by their rules, and the *expense* incurred in case of admission, operates to the exclusion of the most destitute.[37] (Italics in original)

In other words, the Lock Hospital was erected for those members of society who could not afford to pay for the fees that specialist hospitals required for treatment, and for patients who did not have any parish settlement. At the same time we can infer that, after the massive migration to London of people from the countryside as a result of the Industrial Revolution, a considerable number of both men and women would have to go to the Lock gates seeking for relief to obtain a bed for free. The argument of the uniqueness of the Lock Hospital was used to attract funding, but it was not very precise as the Institution was not the only one or the first to provide this kind of attention. For example, Kingsland Hospital had been opened for two centuries only for women with venereal disease, and Guy's and the London Hospital had venereal facilities. Guy's Hospital had been established in 1727, originally intentioned for

---

36 *An Account of the Lock Hospital; to Which is Added an Account of the Lock Asylum, 1837* (The Library, Royal College of Surgeons of England, London), MS0022/3/8.
37 Ibid., MS0022/3/8.

"the incurables", that is, those who had lost all hope of cure. However, it soon developed ward facilities to deal with venereal patients, although the hospital charged admission fees, unlike the other voluntary hospitals. The London Hospital had been founded in 1740 and was situated in the East End to offer venereal care to the suburban poor; in particular, manufacturers, merchant sailors and their wives and children were the beneficiaries of venereal relief. These patients were treated in a separate house following the model of St. Bartholomew's Hospital, but the institution disappeared in 1750.[38]

The reference to prostitutes and to the spread of contagion is veiled in the following lines of the same Annual Report: "It is also worthy of notice, that numbers of these unhappy sufferers if not cured, would be compelled, as their only resource, to linger out their wretched lives, by diffusing their misery in the most rapid progression".[39] It is clear that the unhappy sufferers are prostitutes and that their misery was venereal disease. In the first years of the Lock, prostitutes were not seen as worthy objects of charity, as they were responsible for their own misfortunes, but it was necessary to avoid the spread of disease "in the most rapid progression". Nonetheless, the idea that many respectable married women and innocent children were infected by dissolute husbands was put forward to appeal to the contributor's compassion:

> But indeed many of the pitiable objects of this Charity are, in this respect, free from criminality. Women of irreproachable character become victims to the profligacy of their husbands; nay, infants derive the malady from their parents and nurses; while the vices of such relatives commonly so impoverish their families, as to preclude them from relief except by charity; and it may be affirmed with truth, that of the number of females received within the walls of the hospital, very many of them have not been, very strictly speaking, the vicious and abandoned, but the young, the uninstructed, and the destitute.[40]

38 Siena, *Venereal Disease Hospitals and the Urban Poor: London's Foul Wards 1600–1800*, 217, 220–221.
39 *An Account of the Lock Hospital; to Which is Added an Account of the Lock Asylum, 1837*, MS0022/3/8.
40 ibid..

Introduction: The London Lock Hospital and Asylum

Bearing in mind that the male used to be the sole or the main breadwinner in the family, married women and children with venereal disease had no means to have access to private treatment, especially when the husband was also infected with the foul disease. So, for decent women, the London Lock was the only place they could turn to. A new element appears in the Accounts of the nineteenth century, namely the innocence, ignorance and youth of the female victims, which became a common feature throughout the period and presents a clear difference from the Accounts prior to the last decades of the eighteenth century.

An emblematic symbol of the London Lock Hospital was the Lock Chapel, which had outstanding figures amongst its chaplains and became very popular amongst the middle class, making a very important contribution to the running of the institution. Martin Madan was its founder and it became a huge success, which "quickly boosted the charity's finances".[41]

Madan (1726–1790) was Chaplain to the Charity from 1758 till about 1776, introducing the evangelical element of the last decades of the eighteenth century. He was the son of Colonel Martin Madan, who was a rich county squire, barrister and Member of Parliament. He had graduated in 1746 and during his training in London, he had led a dissolute life, before hearing John Wesley and deciding in 1758 to take holy orders and devote his life to the spread of the Gospel. He was already a Governor of the Foundling Hospital when he proposed himself to become the Chaplain of the London Lock without any salary. His proposal was accepted and he was made a Governor of the Lock. Initially, the South Men's ward was adapted as a place of divine worship, and Madan covered the expense, providing it with a small organ. However, in 1761 the Governors accepted the idea of building a new chapel for 800 people in the garden at the back of the hospital as long as that would not incur any expenditure to the charity.[42] Madan therefore accepted the financial responsibility of building the

---

41   Siena, *Venereal Disease Hospitals and the Urban Poor: London's Foul Wards 1600–1800*, 188.
42   Nicholas Temperley, "The Lock Hospital Chapel and its Music", *Journal of the Royal Music Association* 118, 1 (1993): 48–49.

austere chapel as a simple rectangular building with a pitched roof and five window bays on the long side and galleries. Bromfield negotiated the purchase of an appropriate organ. The chapel was opened in 1762, and Madan preached its opening sermon entitled *Everyman our Neighbour*. The sermon was based on "the biblical lesson that one should love his neighbour as he loves himself".[43] This was clearly a strategy to make an appeal to his middle-class audience to love and help the undeserving poor despite their faults. Patients attended Sunday service entering the Chapel through a separate back door, keeping them apart from the well-to-do community.[44]

It was the tendency for hospitals in the eighteenth century to have chapels. That was the case of the Royal Hospitals and Guy's and the new voluntary hospitals. The model for the London Lock was the Foundling Hospital which had a magnificent Chapel, built with a separate list of subscribers and famous for its preachers and performances of Handel's *Messiah* and other oratorios. It obtained important funds from its impressive congregation by the renting of pews and the sale of tickets for special events.[45] In the case of the Lock Chapel, box pews were hired for one-and-a-half guineas and a seat in the gallery cost three shillings. The music and the sermons of the London Lock became very popular and attracted a huge congregation. Martin Madan's *Collection of Psalms and Hymns* was published and in 1760 he compiled and published his hymn anthology which almost became the only music collection sold at the Lock. Madan became one of the most acclaimed preachers in London, so he spent a lot of time travelling and spent little time with the hospital patients. The truth was that he could not stand the atmosphere in the venereal wards as the awful appearance of the illness in the bodies of the poor was unbearable, even for the best trained members of the medical profession. To substitute for him in some of his tasks, an Assistant Chaplain was appointed, Rev. Thomas Haweis, who remained till 1767, when he left for a rural rectory,

---

43   Siena, *Venereal Disease Hospitals and the Urban Poor: London's Foul Wards 1600–1800*, 191.
44   Innes Williams, *The London Lock: A Charitable Hospital for Venereal Disease, 1746–1952*, 38.
45   Ibid., 37.

and Madan placed in the wards an edition he revised of John Reynold's *Compassionate Address to the Christian World* for the patients to read in his absence. This seems very strange, given that most patients at that time would in all probability have been illiterate, unless Haweis read the text to the patients himself.[46]

But returning to the Lock Hospital music, it groups 127 tunes composed mainly between 1762 and 1792 taken from Madan's *Hymns*, except three. Methodism in its principles and ideas was ever present in the texts, but Madan needed to attract the wealthy and fashionable. This meant giving the Lock music a joyful and positive tone. Theatrical professionals were also strong supporters of the charity, hence the style of the tunes should resemble those of the Italian operas, the oratorios and concerts the audience was familiar with.[47] The Lock Hospital did not have a pool from where to draw a choir; inmates were presumably assumed to look insufficiently inviting to wear a nice uniform and sing before the congregation. Thus, following the Methodist trend of a singing congregation, professional singers were not hired either, and by the beginning of the nineteenth century, a children's choir would lead people attending the service in the Chapel like in the other London churches of the time.[48]

Madan's preoccupation with London's prostitution reached its climax with the publication in 1780 of his book *Thelypaththora or Female Ruin*, where he defends polygamy as the solution for prostitution following the Old Testament. According to the story and to Madan, every man who seduces a young girl should marry her to avoid the downward path of women who sold their bodies. This meant the beginning of the end of his brilliant career and he had to resign the Chaplaincy and retire to Epsom in his last years because of the scandal that ensued.[49]

---

46 Siena, *Venereal Disease Hospitals and the Urban Poor: London's Foul Wards 1600–1800*, 188–189.
47 Temperley, "The Lock Hospital Chapel and its Music", 63–64.
48 Siena, *Venereal Disease Hospitals and the Urban Poor: London's Foul Wards 1600–1800*, 47–48, 54.
49 Innes Williams, *The London Lock: A Charitable Hospital for Venereal Disease, 1746–1952*, 41–42.

The fall of Madan followed that of Bromfield's who had been accused of misappropriation of hospital supplies after retiring from his surgical activity in the Hospital in 1770. A Select Committee was appointed which refused his re-election, so the founding father of the Hospital stopped being a Governor and cut all his ties with the Institution. Both Madan and Bromfield had previously had a confrontation about the duties of the Chaplain, which, in Bromfield's opinion, were very much neglected. This opened the discussion about the patients' religious instruction which furthered the presence of a number of clergymen like Charles de Coetlogon and Thomas Scott: the Charity began to be controlled by a group of Evangelicals after 1780.[50] The moral reform of patients became a fundamental goal of the hospital and began to be used as a key argument in the propaganda appeal to subscribers:

> Among the Patients examples are found of the most ignorant, as well as the most profligate of the human race; and it cannot be expected that they should be met with in places of worship, to receive needful instruction; but the desire of a cure brings them into the Hospital, and there the proper means are used to make them wise unto salvation.[51]

From these lines, we can infer that patients were of the lowest orders of society and not in the habit of going to Church, but the Charity offers the possibility of both a physical and a moral cure which would justify the contributions of middle-class philanthropists to the running of the Institution. The idea, of course, began to be that of "turning patients into useful members of society". However, Evangelicals focused reform mostly on women, and this was the aim behind the foundation of the London Lock Asylum.

The Lock Asylum for the Reception of Penitent Female Patients was established in 1789, and the Chaplain Thomas Scott was the spirit behind this charitable project. It was funded by a different appeal and list

---

50 Siena, *Venereal Disease Hospitals and the Urban Poor: London's Foul Wards 1600–1800*, 198–200.
51 *An Account of the Lock Hospital; to Which is Added an Account of the Lock Asylum, 1837*, MS0022/3/8.

Introduction: The London Lock Hospital and Asylum

of subscribers, and became a key element in the history of the London Lock till its disappearance in the twentieth century.[52] At first, it was open in two small houses in Osnaburg Row, a little street near the Hospital, where up to twenty ladies could be accommodated; later, in 1812, new premises were opened in Knightsbridge and then in Lower Eaton Street because the initial location became small and needed repair. In 1893 the word Asylum was substituted by Rescue Home.[53] The Lock Asylum became very popular, but its degree of success in reforming deviant women was not that high. Only young women who were not assumed to be hardened prostitutes were admitted, and the double standard for men and women which became so popular in the nineteenth century for the bourgeoisie, was clearly behind the aims of this home for fallen women. In other words, men were released from hospital when cured, but women who showed a clear inclination at reform were admitted into the Asylum. As a consequence, it was they who had to be the objects of religious indoctrination and of instruction for a decent working-class job. They were the ones responsible for the spread of illness and sexual promiscuity and the ones who had to be secluded, so as to clean society and to be included in it as pure and non-contaminant members again. The blame was put on one half of the human race ignoring and sanctioning the responsibility of the other. A whole chapter will be devoted to the history and working of the Asylum in the nineteenth century, using materials such as information about asylum inmates, asylum annual reports and accounts and asylum regulations.

In 1842, new buildings were opened for the Hospital and Asylum in Harrow Road, Westbourne Green, comprising

> a Hospital for 50 male patients and 20 females, with the capability to double these numbers, enlarging the wards; an Asylum for 50 females with the possibility to double this number, a Chapel to hold 1,200 persons and separate airing grounds for the male and female patients, and also for the Asylum inmates.[54]

---

52 Innes Williams, *The London Lock: A Charitable Hospital for Venereal Disease, 1746–1952*, 57.
53 *A Short History of the London Lock Hospital and Rescue Home, 1746–1906*, 17–20.
54 Ibid., 23.

New buildings and new wards were added gradually as funds came in, and in 1847 and 1849 respectively a new Chapel – called Christ's Church in 1889 – and the Cambridge or Asylum Wing were built. In 1862, a new building in Dean Street, Soho, was devoted to the Male Branch of the Institution and the Out-patient Department, and the old Hospital became to be known as The Female Hospital, bringing about considerable improvement to the Charity. With the passing of the Contagious Diseases Acts of 1864, 1866 and 1869, and the adaptation of the Hospital to War Office patients, the Prince of Wales or East Wing and the Kinnaird Ward were finally added in 1867 and 1869.[55]

The London Lock Hospital example was followed by a number of voluntary hospitals which were opened in the 18th and 19th centuries throughout the country, like those in Dublin (1792), Glasgow (1805), Manchester and Salford (1819), Liverpool (1834) and Bristol (1870). Some London hospitals used to have lock wards like Guy's Hospital, King's College, Royal Free, St. Bartholomew's, St. Thomas's and Middlesex, but some of them later stopped providing venereal care for foul patients. Venereal wards could also be found in other hospitals and infirmaries in other provinces like Aberdeen Royal Infirmary, Birmingham Queen's Hospital, Edinburgh Royal Infirmary, Exeter and Devon Hospital, Newcastle-on-Tyne Infirmary and Stafford General Infirmary. At the time of the application of the Contagious Diseases Acts of 1864, 1866 and 1869, some government lock hospitals were opened in garrison towns and districts like Aldershot, Chatham, Colchester, Cork, Devonport, Kildare, London, Portsmouth and Shorncliffe.[56] These will be discussed in a later chapter, but this book focuses on the London Lock Hospital and Asylum in the nineteenth century, following Frank Mort's idea that a cultural history of sexuality and its social policing which "evaluates the spatial dimensions of social processes at particular points in time and in more limited settings" remains to be done.[57]

---

55 Ibid., 30.
56 Frederick W. Lowndes, *Lock Hospitals and Lock Wards in General Hospitals* (London: J. & A. Churchill; Liverpool: Adam Holden, 1882), 2, 20–21, 22, 27.
57 Frank Mort, *Dangerous Sexualities: Medico-Moral Politics in England since 1830*, 2nd ed. (Routledge: London and New York, 2000), xxiii.

CHAPTER 2

Fallen Women, Prostitutes and the Treatment of Venereal Disease in the Nineteenth Century

To understand the operations of the London Lock Hospital and Asylum and other similar institutions in the nineteenth century, it is necessary to analyse various aspects connected with women's sexuality and behaviour. According to the ideology of the double spheres, women were identified with the private domain of home and the family as wives and mothers, or unmarried dependants; men, on the other hand, were associated with the public sphere of paid work, politics, and business, and with economic and legal responsibility for their wives and children. Women were dependant, inferior and subordinate to men. As June Purvis states:

> The influence of middle-class domestic ideology in Victorian society helped to create and maintain gender stereotypes. Thus, femininity became identified with domesticity, service to others, subordination and weakness, while masculinity was associated with life in the competitive world of paid work, strength and domination.[1]

Idealised femininity was asexual and chaste. Women were supposed not to know anything about sex before marriage, and they represented the moral strength that contained men's sexual impulse. In other words, and following the double standard model, unchastity, that is, premarital or extramarital sex, was acceptable in men but unpardonable in women, who could fall into serious disgrace. Once married, women were expected to look the other way regarding their husbands' promiscuous sexual life outside marriage; similarly, sex with their husbands was considered as a woman's duty for the

---

1   June Purvis, *A History of Women's Education in England* (Buckingham: Open University Press, 1991), 4.

act of procreation.[2] Woman's nature was defined: the essence of woman was respectability which was connected with dependency, delicacy and frailty; also with subordination, self-sacrifice and appropriate behaviour.[3] All these feminine traits appeared in all the books, manuals, and periodicals that proliferated and supported gender identities based on sex and class. The natural consequence was that all the women who did not conform to this middle-class ideal of femininity and purity, like prostitutes and *fallen women*, were considered deviant.

A woman who fell from her purity could never return to ordinary society, and a woman was in greater danger than a man. In the case of women, "virtue" and "physical chastity" were interchangeable terms, but that did not apply in the case of men. The idea of chastity as the first of woman's virtues depended on two assumptions: the concept of woman's place, and the concept of woman's special nature. The body of a woman was first her father's property and then her husband's; woman's special nature was determined by the fact that her sexual desires were weak or non-existent. All this led to the belief in woman's moral superiority. At the other extreme, working-class women were believed to be sexually active, and the middle class tried to impose their moral values on them.[4]

The images, values and stereotypes used to define femininity for middle-class women were used to support working-class women's lack of femininity. Three quarters of 19th century English women were born into the working classes. For their parents the struggle to keep alive obliterated most other considerations, and everyone in the family had to earn money as soon as they were able.[5] As I pointed out in Chapter 1, premarital sex was common among some sections of the working class throughout the 19th century. Even among the respectable it was often considered unthrifty

---

[2] Linda Mahood, *The Magdalenes: Prostitution in the Nineteenth Century* (London & New York: Routledge, 1990), 4.

[3] Lynda Nead, *Myths of Sexuality: Representations of Women in Victorian Britain* (London: Blackwell, 1988), 28–29.

[4] Sally Mitchell, *The Fallen Angel: Chastity, Class and Women's Reading 1835–1880* (Bowling Green, Ohio: Bowling Green University Popular Press, 1981), x–xiii.

[5] Joan Perkin, *Victorian Women* (Cambridge: Cambridge University Press, 1994), 169.

and unnecessary to marry a girl who had not given evidence of fertility. A large number of illegitimate children born in England were in fact the offspring of common-law unions. These practices were embedded in whole communities. Marriage was not looked on as a liability for a man and a favour for a woman, but as a necessity for their own joint personal survival. Prostitution tended to be viewed as part of women's overall sexual and economic exploitation, due to the restriction of women's entry to employment and born out of sheer economic necessity.[6] As far as the sexual life of the working-class woman was concerned, her attractiveness and self-respect disappeared very soon because of childbirth, suckling, and inadequate diet; due to the sanitary conditions of working-class dwellings, this woman together with her husband and children would have a dirty aspect, their bodies would not smell nicely and they would be infected with lice; they did not know anything about dental hygiene either. The fear of pregnancy and the absence of privacy in a household full of children and lodgers, her husband's violence and drunkenness, debts, miscarriages, the death of some of her children, the unemployment or imprisonment of her husband and his eventual desertion, made her feel anxiety and lose all the excitement about her sexual life.[7]

According to Foucault, sexuality is a historical construct and the nineteenth century was characterised by the description of different sexualities. He uses the concept of "discourse to refer to the set of concepts, values, and practices that define, inform, and justify a set of social relations".[8] As a consequence, different sexualities do not exist outside a particular discourse, and "the history of sexuality is the history of what certain discourses have said about sex". The first time the term *common prostitute* was used was in the Vagrancy Act of 1824 and since then it has been applied to the woman who exchanges sex for money, using her body as a commodity. Prostitution was considered the *Great Social Evil* by Victorians and one form of deviancy;

---

6   Ibid., 178.
7   Fraser Harrison, *The Dark Angel: Aspects of Victorian Sexuality* (London: Sheldon Press, 1977), 176–178.
8   Mahood, *The Magdalenes: Prostitution in the Nineteenth Century*, 6, 8.

it represented a threat to the patriarchal family, as married men committed adultery and the male youth was corrupted. According to the discourses of the time, immorality was increasing in Britain and the general fear focused on one particular form: prostitution.[9] The category of prostitute was not fixed or internally coherent; it could define any woman who transgressed the bourgeois code of morality. The combination of money and the public sphere made the prostitute powerful and independent and these features became a menace to middle-class values. In Lynda Nead's words, "the term *prostitute* is an historical construction which works to define and categorise a particular group of women in terms of sex and class", that is, the term *prostitute* was a label used to identify a working-class woman who sold her sexual favours occasionally or on a permanent basis.[10]

However, prostitution was also defined in terms of disease and ill health that could be spread through contagion. As a consequence, it had to be contained and cured.[11] Prostitutes were the image of public vice and represented a threat to the moral values that lay behind the social organisation of the state and the Empire; they brought chaos and social decay. Prostitution was described as a specifically urban vice; it was associated with the working classes overcrowding the city and polluting it after the Industrial Revolution. Overcrowding was seen as one of the main reasons for prostitution, immorality was associated with poverty, and poverty with the working classes; large families living and sleeping together in one room made chastity a utopia.[12] Nonetheless, there was another definition of the prostitute as a social victim, a hopeless outcast believed to follow a downward path, making her the object of the medical discourse and philanthropy. She became then "a suitable object of charity and compassion" and this idea was appropriated by the London Lock propaganda in the nineteenth century.[13] Images of seduction and the downward path to

---

9   Nead, *Myths of Sexuality: Representations of Women in Victorian Britain*, 93.
10 Ibid., 94–95.
11 Ibid., 120–121.
12 Paula Bartley, *Prostitution: Prevention and Reform in England, 1860–1914* (London & New York: Routledge, 2000), 10.
13 Mahood, *The Magdalenes: Prostitution in the Nineteenth Century*, 55.

destruction appeared frequently in the Accounts for the Lock Hospital and Asylum for the 1820s and 1830s. Thus, in the Account for 1834 we can find the following:

> Young women, having been seduced, deserted and banished from their friends, are frequently left with [sic] any other resource than that of entering the recesses of debauchery; the general consequences of which are increasing wickedness, a ruined constitution, a premature death, and, as far as we can see, everlasting destruction.[14]

With these words the prostitute is presented as a victim and as a consequence an object of compassion, whose end is death and destruction if she is not helped by the Institution.

Most social investigators and reformers identified poverty as the main cause of prostitution. William Tait, one of these middle-class enquirers, divided the causes that led women into prostitution into two kinds, natural and accidental, in his 1841 study *Magdalenism. An Enqiry into the Extent, Causes, and Consequences of Prostitution in Edinburgh*. Among the natural causes were moral failings such as licentiousness, irritability of temper, pride, love of dress, dishonesty, love of property, and indolence; among the accidental were those features of lower-class life, such as seduction, ill-assorted marriages, low wages, want of employment, intemperance, poverty, ill-training, obscene publications, and overcrowded housing.[15] For example, the London Lock Accounts in the 1830s and 1840s tell us about the prostitutes that "they learn extravagance; hence, they sally forth to make [sic] degradations to support the expenses of licentious indulgence".[16] Seduction and the ensuing desertion associated prostitutes with upper-class men, making them the victims in conventional stereotypes like those of flower girls who frequented West End theatres, seamstresses swindled by clients, or servants who had been raped by their masters or their sons. However, stories of seduction of virgins by depraved aristocrats were just part of the

---

14   *Account of the Lock Hospital and Asylum, 1834* (The Library, Royal College of Surgeons of England, London), MS0022/3/8.
15   Judith R. Walkowitz, *Prostitution and Victorian Society: Women, Class and the State* (Cambridge: Cambridge University Press, 1991), 38.
16   *Account of the Lock Hospital and Asylum, 1834*, MS0022/3/8.

myth surrounding the prostitute and her fall, as we shall see later in this chapter, although it might sometimes happen. William Logan, author of *The Great Social Evil; its Causes, Extent, Results and Remedies* (1871) and a temperance reformer, put the emphasis on drink, although he shared William Tait's identification of causes of prostitution. For him, most prostitutes were dependent on gin and narcotics, and public houses had a serious responsibility in inciting male sexual instinct, making both these women and their clients drink to excess. Thereby, they profited from the sale of alcohol, as the existing licensing laws allowed them to stay open all day.[17]

Following the tendency to classification of the nineteenth century described by Foucault, there was a hierarchy of different kinds of women who plied the trade.[18] The most accepted and accurate classification of the time was that of Henry Mayhew in his *London Labour and the London Poor* (1851), where he mentions several categories of these women. He divided prostitutes into six kinds, although he omitted the highest rank of the courtesan. According to him, there were kept mistresses and prima donnas; women living together in well kept lodging houses; women living in low lodging houses; sailors' and soldiers' women; park women; and thieves' women.

The high-class courtesan he did not mention led an upper-class life and could demand huge fees for her services; they used to have protectors and chose them as lovers or changed them when they wished; they lived in houses in fashionable areas and had a great social life in public with the men they favoured. The next in the scale were the kept mistresses who saw their situation as a way of avoiding the dangers of the streets and even had children by their lovers; these women and their offspring had a similar life to that of other decent upper-class women. Prostitutes of lower rank were called prima donnas by Henry Mayhew; they were available at certain fashionable places in London such as parks, theatres and concert

---

17   Bartley, *Prostitution: Prevention and Reform in England, 1860–1914*, 4, 6.
18   Michel Foucault, *The History of Sexuality: Volume I, An Introduction*, trans. Robert Hurley (London: Penguin, 1990), 17–35. The nineteenth century was a time when different forms of human sexuality were analysed and classified.

halls, getting two or three sovereigns (40 to 60 shillings) for sex; they also used to have a male friend who visited them regularly and provided them with part of their needs. The West End prostitutes living in lodgings could exercise their trade securely; they were extravagant and their average earnings were between twenty and thirty pounds a week. Those who lived in lodgings near the Haymarket and in the East End did not fare so well; their earnings varied from three to ten pounds a week, and were known as *convives* and *hunters*. Sailors' and soldiers' women proliferated in areas of London and other major cities where these men could be found; they met their clients at the docks of seaports and in army towns, where they lived in lodgings and did their job in public houses or any other place of public entertainment; they needed to go with many clients and make them drink a great amount of alcohol. Park women, known as *dollymops*, were not professional prostitutes but servant maids, nursemaids, shop girls and milliners who frequented certain recreational places and went occasionally with men and soldiers who accosted them in parks, streets or shops. Finally, thieves' women were the lowest category and were found in the Covent Garden area and later in the Barbican; they lived in streets around Drury Lane and made about sixpence for going with a man.[19]

In contrast, William Acton, an outstanding figure in the medical and social discourses of the time, and an important voice in the Contagious Diseases Acts debate, showed a different view on prostitution. To a certain extent, he contradicted the traditional myth. In his book of 1857, *The Functions and Disorders of the Reproductive Organs in Youth, in Adult Age, and in Advanced Life* he affirms, uncontroversially for the time, that the majority of women lack any kind of sexual feeling, following the tendency of the period. In his other book published the same year, *Prostitution Considered in its Moral, Social and Sanitary Aspects, in London and other Large Cities with Proposals for the Mitigation and Prevention of its Attendant Evils*, of which he wrote a second edition in 1870, he sees the body of the prostitute as the agent of both moral and physical contamination. He advocated the inevitability of prostitution, hence the need for regulation

19 Perkin, *Victorian Women*, 220–228.

to diminish its devastating effects, but I will return to Acton and the Contagious Diseases Acts in the chapter devoted to the London Lock Hospital during the years of their application. He defined prostitution as a physical, moral and social problem, but acknowledged the existence of multiple interpretations of the term according to the different discourses.[20]

Although he shared with the other social investigators the idea that poverty together with certain traits of working-class culture were the main causes of prostitution, he saw the trade as a transitory state.[21] In *Prostitution* he talked about the existence of an open and a clandestine prostitution, and he distinguished two types of women in the business: kept mistresses of higher-class of men, and the working-class prostitutes who walked the streets to do their job. Similarly, he believed that there were women in this class who were not very much depraved, but more respectable and yearning to return to decent society.[22] He questioned the myth of the downward path as he believed that prostitutes, or at least most of them, did not end in destitution and death but by getting married, getting jobs, running their own businesses, or resorting to emigration, so they could move out of the trade. In the chapter entitled "The modern harlot's progress", he mentions the "three vulgar errors about prostitution":

1. That once a harlot, always a harlot
2. That there is no possible advance, moral or physical in the condition of the actual prostitute
3. That the harlot's progress is short and rapid.[23]

---

20 Nina Atwood, *The Prostitute's Body: Rewriting Prostitution in Victorian Britain* (London: Pickering and Chatto, 2011), 25–26.
21 William Acton, *Prostitution Considered in its Moral, Social and Sanitary Aspects, in London and other Large Cities with Proposals for the Mitigation and Prevention of its Attendant Evils* (London: John Churchill, New Burlington Street, 1857b), 64, 73.
22 Atwood, *The Prostitute's Body: Rewriting Prostitution in Victorian Britain*, 26, 28.
23 Acton, *Prostitution Considered in its Moral, Social and Sanitary Aspects, in London and other Large Cities with Proposals for the Mitigation and Prevention of its Attendant Evils*, 52.

This is the view common to most middle-class social reformers, philanthropists, medical men and scientists, and he clearly states the opposite. He believes that most prostitutes had a better life than their working-class sisters, and after more or less four years, were prepared to escape and change their lives. Therefore, he rejected the dramatic opinion that the middle class had about prostitution and recommended regulation to make it a safe and healthy activity. In the light of Acton's ideas, it is clear that there is no system of representation which is totalising, even if they are supported by official or dominant ideologies.

Victorian prostitution happened in most cities in Britain and there were areas where these women used to work and neighbourhoods where they used to live. Most of them were working-class women who had had their first sexual experience with a man of their class on a non-commercial basis, breaking thus the myth of seduction. Their age of initiation was usually sixteen, and their family backgrounds were very similar: most of them had lost one or both parents and the family relations had been frequently disrupted. According to working-class values, they were supposed to support themselves and contribute to the family income. Some of them also came from broken families with a deserted mother or separated parents. After their first fall, these women entered prostitution one or two years later, so they were in their late teens. They remained in the trade till past their mid-twenties, when they became ill or died, or hopefully returned to a respectable working-class life. It seems that most of these women did not have children after they entered prostitution. According to some doctors, some of them were infertile and very few of their offspring survived. Venereal disease must have had an effect on infertility, but most prostitutes with children left them with someone or in the workhouse and employed contraception, abortion and infanticide to avoid the results of their intense sexual activity.[24]

The geographical distribution of prostitutes had very much to do with the employment opportunities open to working-class women. Most prostitutes had been dressmakers, shop assistants, farm workers, barmaids

---

24 Walkowitz, *Prostitution and Victorian Society: Women, Class and the State*, 16–19.

or domestic servants previously. It seems that most of them concentrated in ports and pleasure towns. The lure of London and other important cities was really strong among those from the provinces, as places with an important clientele. However, the concentration of prostitutes in rural and industrial areas was relatively small because stable employment for men and women permitted traditional courtship with premarital sexual relations that led to marriage.[25] Contrary to the general opinion held by both Victorians and modern commentators, middle-class men did not resort to working-class prostitutes; they had their own brothels and recreation places to go. In Victorian Britain there was a clear distinction between the *respectable classes* and the *poor classes*, and the conditions in which prostitutes lived, lacking personal cleanliness and good manners and other middle-class values, made them the object of a working-class clientele.[26]

The street-walker had very little respect for her client who was a man prepared to risk contagion and thus contaminating his wife; he was usually drunk and ready to risk physical violence. He was also prepared to be the object of theft. Prostitutes considered themselves exploited by their male customers and thought it fair to exploit them themselves. The *wages of sin*, as their earnings were known, depended on the rank of prostitute and on the area where she plied her trade.[27] According to the information given by police reports and social investigators, very few prostitutes resided in brothels but frequented them to do their job, although the licensing laws of the second half of the nineteenth century made it more difficult for prostitutes to resort to these places.[28] Brothel-keepers supplemented their earnings with the high rents for prostitutes' rooms, a percentage of the prostitute's wages and the board and lodging of these women. Nonetheless, their main profit was based on the consumption of alcohol by both prostitutes and especially their male clients, as mentioned above.[29]

---

25   Ibid., 22–23.
26   Frances Finnegan, *Poverty and Prostitution: A Study of Victorian Prostitutes in York* (Cambridge: Cambridge University Press, 1979), 67.
27   Ibid., 116.
28   Walkowitz, *Prostitution and Victorian Society: Women, Class and the State*, 24.
29   Finnegan, *Poverty and Prostitution: A Study of Victorian Prostitutes in York*, 109.

Despite all this, most prostitutes met their clients in public houses and other places of entertainment in the neighbourhood where they lived and where working-class customers could be found. They were independent of pimps in most cases, with very few exceptions, like the East End *bullies*. On the whole, Victorian prostitution was a trade organised by women. In fact, most lodging-house keepers were female, and they protected and assisted prostitutes but also had an interest in the prostitutes' activities. There was a strong female subculture in the world of prostitutes; they used to go together and work in couples, which allowed them to commit the petty offences of which they were sometimes accused and to protect each other. There existed group solidarity among these women, but there were also brawls between them over territory. They adopted a similar appearance and they had a dress code which identified them and distinguished them from respectable working-class women. They used conspicuous makeup and imitated their middle and upper-class peers.[30] As far as regulation was concerned, the Vagrancy Act of 1824 has already been mentioned, where the term *common prostitute* was first used, and any woman who behaved "riotously" or "indecently" could be fined or imprisoned. The next law to control prostitution only in London was the Metropolitan Police Act of 1839, where *loitering* and *soliciting* were criminalised and subject to arrest and, if convicted, to a fine that could be increased if the woman was a persistent offender. This law was extended to the rest of England in 1847 with the Towns Police Clauses Act. Only with the Criminal Law Amendment Act of 1885 were important changes brought about. The age of consent for sexual intercourse was raised from 13 to 16 for both sexes, and procurement and forcible detainment of women for the purpose of prostitution were criminalised. Brothels or premises used as such were suppressed and their owners liable to fines and a maximum of three months' imprisonment. Under this new situation, prostitutes could not live or work together and these measures made their lives harder. In 1898, there was a new Amendment to the Vagrancy Act passed, making pimping a criminal offence, but very few

---

30 Walkowitz, *Prostitution and Victorian Society: Women, Class and the State*, 25–28.

pimps were condemned while a great number of women were convicted for "soliciting".[31]

Independently of their image as victims or as agents of sin, prostitutes were seen mainly as the carriers of venereal disease. There were no reliable estimates for the number of prostitutes or for the incidence of venereal disease (VD) in the nineteenth century.[32] Military statistics certainly revealed a high incidence in soldiers and sailors and, as far as the civilian population was concerned, only death rates can give an approximate estimation when the cause of death was revealed as syphilis, although parasyphilitic diseases and congenital syphilis were not identified till later in the period.[33] In any case, syphilis was endemic to Victorian England and it affected both the upper and middle class and the urban poor; it was especially deadly for children during their first year, and contemporary estimates suggest that 10% of the inhabitants of big cities were infected with the illness. It was a very much dreaded ailment as "the peculiar terror of syphilis lay not only in its ghastly symptoms but in the hidden and undetectable nature of its progress".[34]

Venereal diseases are sexually transmitted diseases that can be cured with antibiotics nowadays. The two most important ones are syphilis and gonorrhoea, but also chancroid and venereal warts have an important impact on the population. Syphilis is caused by the bacteria *treponema pallidum*, which do not cause any symptoms in the early stages; it has three stages, with different symptoms each. Primary syphilis appears between 2 to 12 weeks after sexual intercourse with an infected person; a painless red sore can appear on the genitals and also on the mouth and the rectal area,

---

31   J. Laite, *Paying the Price again: Prostitution Policy in Historical Perspective* (2006), accessed May 5, 2008, <http://www.historyandpolicy.org/papers/policy-paper-46.html>, 3–5.

32   E.M. Sigsworth and T.J. Wyke, "A Study of Victorian Prostitution and Venereal Disease" in *Suffer and Be Still: Women in the Victorian Age*, ed. Martha Vicinus (Bloomington & London: Indiana University Press, 1973), 78–79.

33   Walkowitz, *Prostitution and Victorian Society: Women, Class and the State*, 48–49.

34   Mary Wilson Carpenter, *Health, Medicine and Society in Victorian England* (Oxford: ABC Clio, 2010), 72.

and enlarged lymph nodes might be added to the symptoms; chancres can heal in between 3 and 6 weeks, but if the infection is not treated, the disease continues to its second stage. Secondary syphilis usually begins after a few weeks and a few months after the primary stage; the bacteria enters the blood and spreads through the body causing various symptoms like rash (small red spots), fever, headache, loss of appetite, weight loss, sore throat, muscle aches, joint pain, a generally ill feeling and enlarged nymph nodes. The rash can also appear on the palms and the sores, the trunk, arms and legs; condylomata (grey or wart-like patches of skin) can appear on humid areas around the mouth, anus and vagina; the liver, kidneys and eyes can be affected, and the lesions are very contagious, sometimes even causing meningitis; these symptoms will also disappear, but without treatment the illness develops to its tertiary stage. Late or tertiary syphilis can develop after a latent stage and its symptoms can appear years later damaging the eyes, large blood vessels, heart, bones and central nervous system (neurosyphilis); other symptoms are loss of memory, mental function problems, problems with walking and balance, with the bladder, vision, and impotence and loss of feeling in the legs.[35] This last symptom was called "a sore leg" in the eighteenth century.

Gonorrhoea is caused by the bacterium *Neisseria gonorrhoeae* and is transmitted through bodily fluid in all types of sex (vaginal, oral and anal). About 60 per cent of women and 10 per cent of men do not develop any symptoms; when the symptoms appear, the infection can affect the vagina, cervix, urethra, rectum, throat and the eye. In men, a pus-stained discharge from the penis and pain on passing urine can occur and the infection can spread to the prostate and testicles; in women, the infection can cause pelvic inflammatory disease (PID) and as a result provoke sterility. Untreated women can pass the illness on to the baby in childbirth affecting its eyesight if left uncured.[36]

---

35 "Syphilis", accessed August 8, 2012, <http://kidshealth.org/parent/infections/std/syphilis.html#cat20046>.
36 "Gonorrhoea: Symptoms and Treatments", accessed March 3, 2009, <http://www.ivillage.co.uk/print/0,9688,665001,00.html>.

Chancroid is caused by the bacteria *Haemophilus ducreyi* and produces ulcers of the genitals. In men, swollen, painful lymph glands (inguinal buboes) may appear on the groin area. The symptoms usually appear between 4 and 10 days of contact; the ulcer – sometimes called soft chancre because it is soft to the touch – is a tender elevated bump that becomes a pus-filled, open sore with eroded or ragged edges. Chancroid is often asymptomatic in women.[37]

Finally, venereal warts or genital warts are growths or bumps contracted through sexual intercourse and caused by certain types of the human papillomavirus (HPV). They appear in and around the vagina or anus and on the cervix in females; in males they can be found on the penis, scrotum, groin or thigh. Sometimes they cluster together and acquire the form of a cauliflower. The changes in the cervix that happen in the case of women can lead to cancer and in men cancer of the penis or the anus can be developed. This is the only venereal disease that has no treatment, but the warts can be removed with freezing or laser.[38]

In the middle ages, gonorrhoea was seen as the fermentation of the sperm or as the result of an ulcer in the urethra, so it was believed to affect men, and the treatment was bandages for the penis and the introduction of a live flea in the urethra. Although most writers did not recognise the incidence of the ailment in women, they were considered as the source of the infection. Syphilis seems to have appeared in Europe around 1495, and some historians attribute it to the return to Europe of the expedition of Christopher Columbus from the South-American continent. In the sixteenth century, some writers saw gonorrhoea and chancroid as symptoms of syphilis, as they were confused by the similarity of the parts of the body and organs affected and by the fact that transmission was produced during sexual intercourse. They did realise that syphilis affected both men and women, but the medical literature centred on men.[39]

---

37 "Chancroid", accessed March 8, 2009, <http://www.idph.state.il.us/public/hb/hbchancroid.htm>.
38 "Genital Warts", accessed March 3, 2009, <http://kidshealth.org/parent/inefections/std/genital_warts.html#cat20046>.
39 Mary Spongberg, *Feminising Venereal Disease: The Body of the Prostitute in Nineteenth Century Medical Discourse* (London: Macmillan, 1997), 17–19.

In the middle ages, leprosy was considered the illness of corruption and depravity, the leper's body was a social text of moral decay, and the word "lock" was associated with its victims. This reading is coincident with Susan Bordo's notion of the body as "a text of culture", to which I will return in other parts of the book; cultural notions connected with ideas about health and illness were seen as displayed on the lepers' bodies. The representation at this time of venereal disease as a personification of a female form had also its cultural implications, as it was believed that women were the contaminators, spreading the "foul" disease. Both leprosy and syphilis had been related to certain humoral disorders in women, and it was believed that women could contaminate men with these venereal diseases while they remained clean and immune to them.[40] The word "lock" had different historical and social implications. The term was on the one hand associated with the fact that patients were literally "locked up", that is, segregated because of the contagious nature of the illness they were suffering – this was the case of leprosy and later of venereal disease – and, on the other, it was believed that the term was derived from the French *les locques*. These were the dressings or rags with which leprous and poxy patients covered their sores; they had to deposit them in a receptacle outside the doors before entering a church.[41] It can therefore be inferred that venereal disease became to be considered as an ailment similar to leprosy, in the sense of the physical decay and moral corruption that it implied.

---

40 Susan Bordo introduces the concept of the body as a "text of culture" because "different bodies are assigned different locations, are represented differently in prevailing cultural codes, and are accorded different authority as producers of knowledge", quoted in Vincent B. Leitch, ed., *The Norton Anthology of Theory and Criticism* (New York and London: W-W Norton & Company, 2001), 2240–2241. One way in which the body becomes a producer of culture is through the binaries purity/pollution or healthy/corrupted that could be applied both to the lepers' and the venereally diseased bodies. Bodies as such can then produce cultural and social knowledge in the Foucauldian sense of the word. Bodies can similarly produce knowledge through gender, and this is particularly relevant to notions associated with the workings of the London Lock.

41 Robert Lees, "The 'Lock Wards' of Edinburgh Royal Infirmary", *British Journal of Venereal Disease* 37, 3 (1961): 187.

At the same time and due to the contagious nature of venereal disease, those suffering from syphilis or gonorrhoea were seen as having to be isolated in order to avoid the spread of an illness which was associated with the lack of morals and sexual laxity of the undeserving poor.

In the eighteenth century there was a widespread belief that gonorrhoea could have different forms which could or could not lead to syphilis. One form was simple gonorrhoea which appeared in a spontaneous way and was non-venereal; then, there were two forms of venereal gonorrhoea which were the result of impure intercourse. The first form of venereal gonorrhoea had to do with intercourse during menstruation, vaginal discharges or with inflammatory states of the vagina; it was unpleasant, but not contagious. True gonorrhoea was infectious and became syphilis if not treated. John Hunter, an eminent Scottish surgeon, anatomist, physiologist and pathologist contributed to the unity theory about venereal disease in his volume *On the Venereal Disease* published in 1786. Hunter became a very much respected authority and following his ideas the "unity of the virus" theory was prevalent in England till the 1840s. As a result of an experiment, he thought that gonorrhoea and syphilis were the same poison; he inoculated the glans penis – some say his own, others say probably a patient's – with the discharge of another patient suffering from gonorrhoea. After ten days a syphilitic chancre appeared, in all probability because the donor had the two infections, but this fact allowed him to assert that the unity theory was correct and that the two diseases could not coexist.[42] Hunter made a distinction between true and spontaneous gonorrhoea and between a venereal and a simple clap, but he failed to describe their different symptoms.[43] He made many mistakes –such as denying the existence of hereditary syphilis, he did not think that syphilis could be transmitted through the blood or that a suckling infant could get it – and he believed that secondary symptoms were not contagious. He even denied that the brain or viscera could

---

42 Innes Williams, *The London Lock: A Charitable Hospital for Venereal Disease, 1746–1952*, 8.
43 The "clap" and the "itch" were names given to venereal disease in the eighteenth and nineteenth centuries, particularly to syphilis.

be affected during the tertiary stage, delaying the investigations about the true nature of the disease as it progressed.[44]

The unity theory was the object of debate in the 1830s. It had first been contested in 1793 by Benjamin Bell, a Scottish surgeon, in his *Treatise on Gonorrhoea and Lues Venerea*. His statements corresponded with clinical observation and he concluded that syphilis and gonorrhoea had two different clinical pictures and responded in different ways to treatment. He believed that inoculation experiments could be valid only if they were repeated with a number of patients, so that the conclusions could be clinically proved. Richard Carmichael, Superintendent of the Dublin Lock Hospital, only contributed to the confusion in 1814, subdividing venereal disease into four classes, each of which was produced by a different poison and produced different effects. However, he was right in asserting that syphilis could appear in a variety of manifestations. Finally, John Abernethy, a pupil of Hunter, contributed to the debate during the same period but maintained that the division between "true syphilis" and "pseudo-syphilis" was valid and that only some secondary symptoms were in fact syphilitic.[45]

Nonetheless, it was not until Philippe Ricord published his *Traité Practique sur les Maladies Vénériennes* in 1838 that doctors could distinguish between gonorrhoea and syphilis, and the three stages in the latter be clearly established. He based his discoveries on empirical research and human experiments. Since then, British medical authorities have known that syphilis was an infectious disease produced by sexual intercourse and that within 24 days of contagion an indurated sore would appear; after six to eight weeks secondary syphilis would follow accompanied by a fever, depression, pain in the joints and limbs and a generalised eruption. Tertiary syphilis could appear several years after the first infection, with sores and bone disorders, and other fatal symptoms that affected the liver, lungs, brain and muscles, accompanied by a generally debilitating

44 Spongberg, *Feminising Venereal Disease: The Body of the Prostitute in Nineteenth Century Medical Discourse*, 25.
45 Ibid., 31.

effect. Ricord also identified gonorrhoea as "a purulent inflammation of the mucous membranes" that affected the urethra in men and the vagina in women. He thought that it was a mild disease in men and that women hardly suffered from it. The same as many other medical authorities of the time, he believed that women's discharges and secretions could contaminate men with the venereal or non-venereal poison, especially favoured by the consumption of alcohol, a rich diet – he mentioned asparagus and oysters – and excessive sexual activity.[46] However, he did not realise that gonorrhoea could reach women's internal reproductive organs and cause pelvic inflammatory disease (PID). Ricord also introduced the use of the speculum "to look into the vagina and see symptoms not visible on manual pelvic examination".[47]

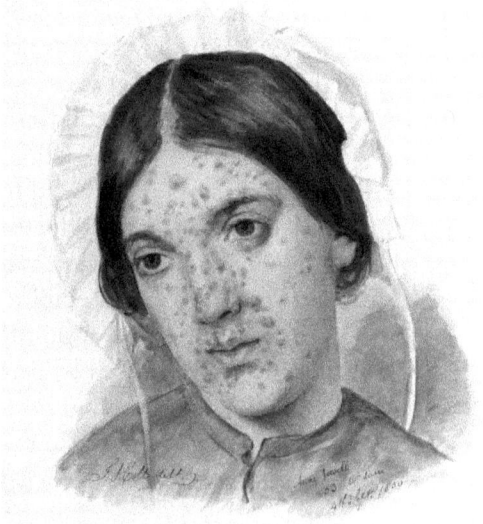

Picture of Anne Sewell, 4th September 1850, Portrait by J. Holt, Patients' Records, the Library, Royal College of Surgeons of England, MS0022/6/6.

46 Walkowitz, *Prostitution and Victorian Society: Women, Class and the State*, 50–51, 53–54.
47 Wilson Carpenter, *Health, Medicine and Society in Victorian England*, 83.

Fallen Women, Prostitutes and the Treatment of Venereal Disease

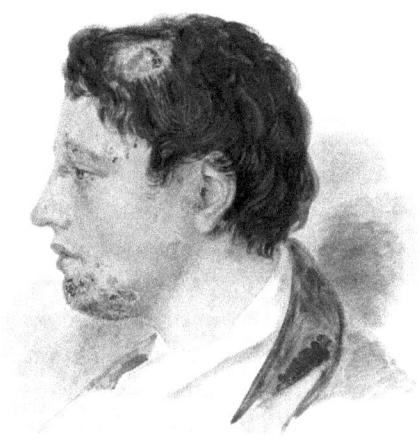

Picture of William Bentley, 23rd April 1850, Portrait by J. Holt, Patients' Records, the Library, Royal College of Surgeons of England, MS0022/6/6.

Venereal disease was represented in the figure of the prostitute in the nineteenth century, who was seen as the source of contagion both of the physical and the social body. This idea was disseminated in many of the Annual Reports of the London Lock. For example, in the Account for 1834 we can read:

> Moreover, if we consider the influence of such women on population, and the health of the people; and on the conduct of children to their parents, and husbands to their wives; and that commonly the seducers of virtuous young women (whose conduct is so generally and justly execrated) are trained up for such seductions in the company of the licentious; we may, without exaggeration, assert, that a common prostitute is an evil in a community not dissimilar to that of a person infected with the plague; who, miserable in himself, is daily communicating the contagion to others, that will propagate still wider the fatal malady.[48]

48 *Account of the Lock Hospital and Asylum, 1834*, MS0022/3/8.

The language of illness and contagion is present in these words together with notions of corruption, depravity and social evil. I have already mentioned that doctors like Hunter, and Acton later, thought that discharges in women could cause venereal disease in men as a kind of allergic reaction to impure intercourse so that this notion implied that women's bodies were pathological bodies if not innately diseased bodies; there were even doctors like Parker or Holmes Coote who talked about the spread of venereal disease like a catarrah. The more the body was used to disease the more immune it became to it, and in the case of venereal disease this idea could be applied to prostitutes. The fact that many women did not show any signs of the foul disease caused panic among the medical profession as they thought it was really dangerous to risk contagion with these women; at the same time, doctors were not very familiar with the different vaginal discharges, so confusion was prevalent.[49] Some went even further by suggesting that not only prostitutes but decent women could spread the disease, and according to Walkowitz, "by designating all women as potential pollutants of men and reservoirs of infection" this idea "invoked instead a more general hostility and dread of females and female 'nature'".[50] Therefore the vagina was the place where the disease originated and from which it spread, especially because of its irritant character; as a result, in the early decades of the nineteenth century, the female body began to be medicalised as both a sexed and a diseased body.

Medicine started to be preventive and environmental, and medical policing also became a characteristic of British society. Doctors believed that some ailments had external causes, so they could be controlled and eradicated. In the case of venereal disease, it was the prostitute's body that had to be controlled, and this was one of the arguments for regulation that I will discuss later in the book.[51] By the middle of the nineteenth century, miasma theory had become very popular. This theory of disease was based on the belief that putrid matter could be found in places like marshes,

---

49   Spongberg, *Feminising Venereal Disease: The Body of the Prostitute in Nineteenth Century Medical Discourse*, 26, 32.
50   Walkowitz, *Prostitution and Victorian Society: Women, Class and the State*, 56.
51   Spongberg, *Feminising Venereal Disease: The Body of the Prostitute in Nineteenth Century Medical Discourse*, 35–36.

drains, sewers and cemeteries, and was responsible for the contagion of many diseases; this model served the medical profession to link prostitution with the "foul" disease. In that sense, the prostitute's bodily discharges were identified with miasma that contaminated clean and pure society. This led to the blurring of the boundaries between sexual promiscuity and immorality, and poverty, which was associated with filth and squalor, was seen as the result of depravity and morally contagious.[52]

However, there was one more form of venereal disease, congenital or hereditary syphilis, which had been mostly ignored throughout the nineteenth century. According to Mary Wilson Carpenter, it was Jonathan Hutchinson who identified the illness in the 1880s establishing a diagnosis when two of the three elements in his triad could be identified as symptoms in the patient: interstitial keratitis, or inflammation of the cornea, notched or incisor teeth and deafness. This method allowed him to identify a syphilitic infection even if it appeared in the sufferer's twenties or thirties. In the same period, Alfred Fournier believed that syphilis was transmitted through the father's semen, transforming the male body in the carrier of inherent degeneracy instead of the female. In other words, the disease could be transmitted by the sperm of an infected man when it was united with the woman's ovum in the act of procreation, although we now know that the foetus can be also infected by the placenta or by contact with a syphilitic lesion at the moment of birth. Fournier also discovered that *tabes dorsalis* – an infection of the spinal cord which produces pain in the trunk and legs – incontinence and impotence could be attributed to tertiary syphilis, and that motor paralysis and insanity were also symptoms of the last stage.[53] Nevertheless, congenital syphilis had already been described in the same terms almost two decades earlier in Alexander Bruce's *An Epitome of the Venereal Diseases being a Succinct Account of the Well Established and More Important Facts to these Diseases* (1868).[54]

52   Ibid., 53–55.
53   Wilson Carpenter, *Health, Medicine and Society in Victorian England*, 88.
54   Alexander Bruce was Fellow of the Royal College of Surgeons, Assistant Surgeon to the Westminster Hospital and Lecturer on Anatomy in the Medical School. In the title of the treatise appears the sentence "Designed for the use of students attending

The identification of congenital syphilis had very important moral and social consequences in the last decades of the nineteenth century. After the passing of the Matrimonial Causes Act of 1857, women had been able to allege the fact that they had been infected by their husbands to ask for divorce. The Act established that men could obtain the divorce just on the grounds of adultery; however, wives had to prove that they had been victims of an additional offense like bigamy, incest, cruelty or desertion. Cases of venereally diseased wives in court put forward the idea that men were polluting decent women, contesting the notion that women were the repositories of venereal disease and the ones who spread the illness. So it was the sexual misconduct of men that brought these disorders to the sanctuary of the home, making husbands abusive and cruel to their wives as a result of adultery.[55] Many men contracted venereal disease before marriage as they satisfied their sexual appetites with prostitutes to keep their women clean and pure, and many innocent brides were infected by their husbands. Doctors also contributed to the ignorance of these women, by collaborating with these men in concealing the real situation from them, although in the 1880s and 1890s manuals began to proliferate warning about the risk of women giving birth to a syphilitic infant.[56]

Hospital Out-Patient Practice", and it was published by the medically respected firm of H.K. Lewis, of Gower Street, London, at the price of one shilling. It is clear that his aim was the instruction of medical students. He states that "Syphilis may be transmitted to the foetus from either parent" and that "A child affected with syphilis is usually small and sickly, and usually about the 4th or 6th week shews some evidence of its inherited cachexia [...] The permanent teeth are generally small, stunted and peggy in form, of a bad colour; the central incisors are deeply notched [...] Subsequently, the child will be liable to a specific form of inflammation of the cornea (interstitial keratitis), often accompanied by deafness". He also describes other symptoms associated with syphilis, and describes those of the triad identified by Hutchinson.

55 Gail Savage, "'The Wilful Communication of a Loathsome Disease': Marital Conflict and Venereal Disease in Victorian England", *Victorian Studies* 34, 1 (1990): 49–50.
56 Wilson Carpenter, *Health, Medicine and Society in Victorian England*, 89–90.

Fallen Women, Prostitutes and the Treatment of Venereal Disease 47

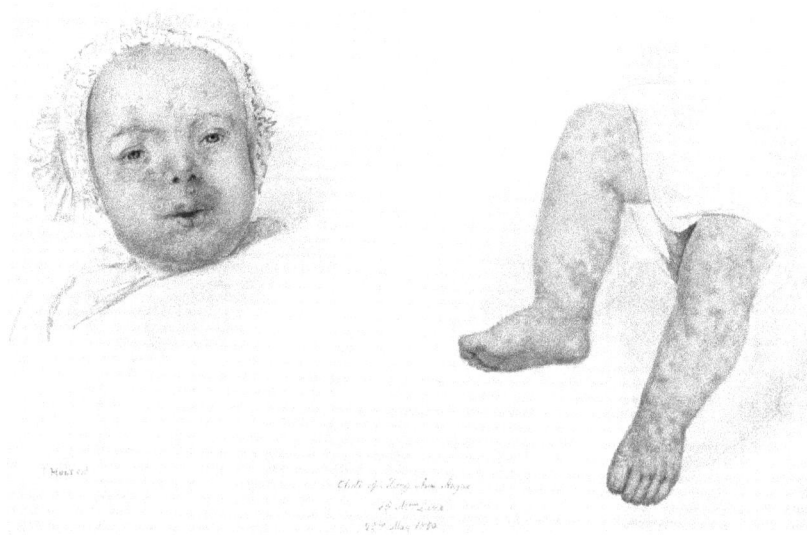

Picture of the child of Mary Ann Agnes, 2nd May 1850, Portrait by J. Holt, Patients' Records, the Library, Royal College of Surgeons of England, MS0022/6/6.

As far as treatment was concerned, it was based on the theory of humours – already mentioned in Chapter 1 – of the classic Greek and Roman literature; in particular, Hippocrates and Galen had believed that illnesses developed because of the internal disturbance of humours. Therefore, treatments tried to restore the different humours to balance. For example syphilis was thought to produce an excess of phlegm, so it was important to make the patient expel it, and for this substances like sarsaparilla and mercury were used.[57] Prevention was not very common, but it seems that prostitutes used oil in the vagina before intercourse, and both men and women used alcoholic and astringent solutions and caustics to destroy the venereal poison after intercourse.[58]

The perception of venereal disease changed deeply from the eighteenth to the nineteenth centuries. A familiarity with the illness can be inferred in

57   Wilson Carpenter, *Health, Medicine and Society in Victorian England*, 75, 77.
58   Walkowitz, *Prostitution and Victorian Society: Women, Class and the State*, 51.

the different books, articles in periodicals and advertisements for remedies in newspapers which became very popular among the literate in the eighteenth century. Literarily as in Defoe's *Roxana* and Smollett's *Roderick Random*, or visually as in Hogarth's series of engravings entitled *Marriage-à-la-Mode* and *Harlot's Progress*, venereal disease figures at some point and the very well-known consequences of the mercurial treatment usually appear, like salivation or loosening teeth. Throughout the eighteenth century around one hundred books and pamphlets were published on venereal disease, most of them by quacks. Sometimes, there was a light-hearted and frivolous attitude towards venereal disease in newspapers of the time, like the *Gentleman's Magazine* and *The Tatler*; this can be seen from the words employed to name it, like *claps* or *French illness*, and it was clearly associated with prostitution.[59]

However, in the nineteenth century, although it was believed that syphilis and gonorrhoea had spread as a consequence of the Napoleonic Wars, the tolerance towards the illness disappeared. Venereal disease was now considered sinful and degrading. Newspaper advertisers grew wary of naming it directly, preferring euphemisms such as *certain disorders*, *certain insidious diseases*, *a few prevailing diseases frequently contracted in a moment of intoxication* – intoxication meaning, of course, sexual intercourse – or *that cruel disease, which is so dreadful a scourge for illicit pleasure*. With the new moral code of the middle classes, the allusions to the ailment which had been clear and ironic in the previous century, even when talking about the symptoms, became obscure in the Victorian era.[60] However, it becomes clear from the advertisements in nineteenth century newspapers that syphilis was the main object of concern, and a familiarity with its different stages and symptoms can be discerned. Most private doctors or quacks announcing their treatments here were against the most common mercurial methods, which were still prevalent in lock hospitals

---

59   A. Fessler and R. Sharpe, "Advertisements on the Treatment of Venereal Diseases in the Eighteenth and Nineteenth Centuries", *British Journal of Venereal Disease* 23, 3 (1947): 125.
60   A. Fessler, "Advertisements on the Treatment of Venereal Disease and the Social History of Venereal Disease", *British Journal of Venereal Disease* 25, 2 (1949), 85, 87.

and wards and caused the most dreadful and conspicuous side-effects. It seems that the main ingredient of the medicines, pills, and drops they offered, like Dr. Cullen's scarlet pills or Dr. Hoffmann's botanical pills, was sarsaparilla; some of these products had a preventive effect and could be applied to both syphilis and gonorrhoea. Secrecy and discretion were offered in these advertisements so as to comply with the moral standards of the time.[61] Special arrangements for female patients were offered. These extracts from advertisements published in the nineteenth century to cure all kinds of patients from the poison of venereal disease which tainted their bodies and blood illustrate all this:

> By the efficacy of Dr. Boerhaave's infallible red pills, (4s. 6d. only per box), persons of either sex (assisted by the invaluable copious directions therewith given) are enabled to eradicate effectually a certain insidious disease, and to facilitate the recovery of health, with ease and safety, certainty and secrecy, in a few days. (*The Lancaster Gazette* of Nov. 27, 1813)

> Cubebs with sarsaparilla, & C. Stirlings Rees' Essence – The vast and increasing sale, from the recommendation of the highest medical characters, as well as those who have experienced its salubrious and beneficial effects, [...] it being the most safe and effectual remedy ever discovered for the cure of Gonorrhoea, Gleets, Seminal Weakness, Strictures, Whites, Pains of the Loins, Kidnies [sic], Gravel, irritation of the Bladder, Urethra and all Disorders of the Urinary Passages, frequently performing a perfect cure in the short space of three or four days. It contains, in a highly concentrated state, all the efficacious parts of the Cubeb, chemically combined with Sarsaparilla, and other choice alternatives, which render it invaluable to those afflicted with secondary Syphilitic symptoms, Ulcers, Pimples, Blotches, Scorbutic Eruptions, Glandular Swellings, and all other diseases arising from a tainted or impure state of the blood. In cases of debility, both local and general, tabes dorsalis, wasting, impotence, and nervous depression of the spirits, it has been taken with the most decided benefit. [...] The most delicate female may take it with perfect safety. It is an excellent substitute for mercury. (*The Blackburn Alfred* of Nov. 6, 1833)[62]

---

61 A. Fessler, "Leaflets on the Treatment of Venereal Diseases of the Early Nineteenth Century", *British Journal of Venereal Disease* 22, 2 (1946): 85–86.

62 Fessler and R. Sharpe, "Advertisements on the Treatment of Venereal Diseases in the Eighteenth and Nineteenth Centuries", 126, 127.

Sarsaparilla and Guaiacum were believed to have the principles to combat the symptoms of venereal disease, as people believed that the illness originated in South American land. Guaiacum was grown in the West Indies and it caused profuse sweating but it did not have any other effects; it probably did not cure the disease and hardly had any impact on it. Sarsaparilla became very popular as a home remedy. These two remedies were very much used, even by medical authorities like the Manchester Surgeon John Lignum. He published his *Treatise on Venereal and Syphilitic Diseases; Containing Plain and Practical Directions for the Effectual Cure of all Degrees of the above Complaints; with Observations on the Uses and Abuses of Mercury Intended for the Instruction of General Readers* in 1819. The book was sold in his dispensary in Manchester, but also at Simpkin & Marshall Stationers' Court in London and all other booksellers in the United Kingdom; it was directed at the general public and, apart from describing the symptoms of the different forms of the "foul" disease and the effects of the mercurial treatment, he includes two recipes for readers based on Sarsaparilla, the Lisbon Diet Drink and Decoction of Sarsaparilla, which read as follows:

> Lisbon Diet Drink
> Or compound Decoction of Sarsaparilla. Take of the root of Sarsaparilla, sliced and bruised, six ounces: bark of the root of Sasafras, shavings of Guaiacum Wood, liquorice root bruised, each one ounce; Mezereon, three drachms, distilled water ten pints. Macerate in the water, with a gentle heat, the Sarsaparilla, Sasafras, Guaiacum, and liquorice, for six hours; then boil it down to five pints, adding towards the end of the boiling, the Mezereon, and strain the liquor. A gill to be taken four times a day.
>
> Decoction of Sarsaparilla
> Take of sliced Sarsaparilla root, six ounces, Distilled Water, four quarts: Digest for two hours in a moderate heat, then take out the Root and bruise it; when bruised, put it back into the same liquor; boil down to two quarts, then press out and strain the decoction.[63]

---

63   John Lignum, *Treatise on Venereal and Syphilitic Diseases; Containing Plain and Practical Directions for the Effectual Cure of all Degrees of the above Complaints; with Observations on the Uses and Abuses of Mercury Intended for the Instruction of General Readers* (Manchester: T. Rogerson, 1819), 54.

Upper- and middle-class gentlemen visited these *advertising doctors* or they could write to them to obtain the remedy as long as they paid for it, receiving the medicine and the "Book of Instructions" with it if they knew the diagnosis. Another way of acquiring the cure was by buying it at any of the shops and premises that could be found in all towns and cities. The scarce treatment facilities made quack doctors proliferate at least until 1916 when the state took control of the treatment of venereal disease of everyone infected, both rich and poor.[64] When a regular doctor was needed, gentlemen used to go to a surgeon, who was thought to be the appropriate kind of professional to treat venereal disease; physicians would only intervene in difficult cases, and of course apothecaries would dispense many of the drugs demanded.

The main treatment for syphilis was mercury in different forms: pills, ointment, vapour bath or injections from the 1860s onwards. As noted, the side-effects of mercury were quite nasty like extreme salivation, loss of teeth and hair, and pain in the teeth and bones; the long-run effects were even more serious. In the first decades of the nineteenth century, many doctors began to be in favour of "the simple method", that is, rest, cleanliness and a supervised diet for the treatment of primary syphilis. Also other treatments were introduced, like those mentioned by Pearson, who was Surgeon to the London Lock between 1782 and 1818; he alluded to more innovative treatments like sulphuric and nitric acids, and iodide of potassium. It has been already mentioned that most doctors did not distinguish between syphilis and gonorrhoea, which was not their object of concern. Nonetheless, gonorrhoea occurred obviously both in women and men, the most extended treatment being the use of irrigation, lotions and ablutions.[65] But treatments evolved as medicine progressed, and in the *Pharmacopeia* of 1887 of the London Lock Hospital for example, we find a description of the different treatments used at the time, which include "balnea", like

---

64 A. Fessler, "Advertisements on the Treatment of Venereal Disease and the Social History of Venereal Disease", 87.
65 T.J., Wyke, "Hospital Facilities for, and Diagnosis and Treatment of, Venereal Disease in England, 1800–1870", *British Journal of Venereal Disease* 49, 1 (1973): 81–82.

"the continuous hot bath", "mercury vapour bath" and "alkaline bath"; "causticae", "collunaria", "decoctum", "gargarismata", "haustus", "injectiones pro vagina" like "injectio aluminis", "injectio astringens", "injectio boracis", "injectio plumbi", "injectio plumbi cum belladonna", "injectio plumbi cum opio" and "injectio zinci cum alumina"; "injections pro urethra", "linimentum", "lotiones", "misturae", "olea", "pilulae", "pulveres" and "unguenta". The same authoritative volume describes an "Ordinary Diet" and "Rules for inunction of mercurial ointments", "Directions for treatment of scabies with sulphur ointment", and "Rules for using the injection". This proves, however, that mercury was still very much in use into the last decades of the nineteenth century.[66]

Nonetheless, it was not till the beginning of the twentieth that new discoveries of various kinds led to the effective cure of venereal disease. In 1905, Fritz Schaudinn and Erich Hoffmann found a method to see the spiral-shaped bacteria *Treponema pallidum* under the microscope, and in 1906 August von Wasserman discovered a blood test for syphilis. When Paul Ehrlich realised that an arsenical compound, later called Salvarsan, was effective to kill the bacteria, a real treatment began to work for people under the foul disease, but it was quite difficult to use and it took quite a long time. Only with the advent of antibiotics and the use of penicillin – also called the magic bullet – in the 1940s could venereal disease be eventually eradicated.[67]

As far as patients receiving treatment in the London Lock Hospital in the second half of the eighteenth century and the first years of the nineteenth are concerned, surviving records show that more men were treated than women, although the figures were balanced by the bigger presence of women in workhouse infirmaries. The Lock Hospital admitted patients only once, and it kept this practice during the nineteenth century as "it has long been known that no person is readmitted, on any recommendation whatever, who has been discharged for irregularity, or has again

---

66 *Pharmacopeia in Use at the Male and Out-Patient Department of the London Lock Hospital* (London: Adlard and Son, Bartholomew Close, 1887), 1–39.
67 Wilson Carpenter, *Health, Medicine and Society in Victorian England*, 74.

received the infection";[68] it seems that the London Lock was particularly important for the itinerant poor that had migrated from the countryside to London, and had contracted venereal disease. Patients were treated for free at the beginning, but after 1760, the Lock authorities began to charge parish officers for sending their paupers (two guineas per patient). The Lock also accepted patients who had travelled a long distance from parishes outside London for a fee and those who did not have any parish settlement in London. According to Siena, the Lock started to charge fees to parishes, so as to stop them sending patients they ought to have looked at parish expense.[69]

The only case books of the London Lock Hospital that have survived are those of John Pearson (1798–1799) and John Ritchie (1813–1814). John Pearson (1758–1826) was elected House Surgeon to the London Lock Hospital and served the Institution for almost forty years. As stated above, Pearson tried different substances like corrosive sublimate, but he found calomel and mercury more effective, using them as an ointment; he also used nitric acid, and describes all his experiments in his book *Observations on various items of Materia Medica used in the Treatment of Lues Venerea* of 1800.[70] Pearson talks about 86 female patients who were quite young (average age 23.3 years) and he mentions several cases of gonorrhoea; most of them were single and probably prostitutes, contradicting the fund-raising literature which stressed the presence of married women and children. However, according to the entries for 1824 I found in the Lock Asylum Committee minutes – written by the Matron in all probability who at the time was a Mrs. Martha Sterling – the average age of inmates was 18.1, being 24 the age of the eldest, and 10 the age of the youngest. This change in the figures can be attributed to the fact that only a small group of women with a clear inclination at reformation and docility were admitted into the

---

68   *An Account of the Lock Hospital; to Which is Added an Account of the Lock Asylum, 1837* (The Library, Royal College of Surgeons of England, London), MS0022/3/8.
69   Siena, *Venereal Disease Hospitals and the Urban Poor: London's Foul Wards 1600–1800*, 225–233.
70   Innes Williams, *The London Lock: A Charitable Hospital for Venereal Disease, 1746–1952*, 54.

Lock Asylum; on the other hand, there was a tendency at the time among middle-class reformers to believe that the younger the women the easier to indoctrinate and save them from a life of degradation. In fact, one of the girls was only ten years old, clearly a child according to all the standards of the age – the age of consent being then thirteen.[71]

Both male and female patients had resorted to self-treatment or private treatment before entering the hospital and after suffering from the "foul" disease for several months, sometimes years. Following Ritchie's notes which cover a smaller sample (only twenty-one men), the average age of male patients was over twenty-eight years. Therefore, they were older than their female counterparts, and they suffered mainly from secondary or tertiary syphilis. But there was no clear case of gonorrhoea and some were infected with chancroid. In both casebooks the date when the patient thought that he or she had contracted venereal disease was recorded; for both doctors this information was essential for treatment. Most male patients had endured the ailment for longer than women, and waiting lists were not infrequent, as at some periods during the eighteenth century there were no available beds. Admission was delayed from about two weeks on average to two months, and applicants were advised to attend every week to see if there were any new vacancies, having then to ask the governors who had nominated them for help.[72] Once admitted, both casebooks reveal that patients remained in the hospital for the time of the salivation treatment with mercury, which remained the main remedy at this time. They were prepared for the procedure for a few days and then suffered the salivating process for about forty days and left immediately or stayed for a brief period before being discharged. Other forms of treatment at the London Lock in those days included the bougie – thin cylinder of rubber, plastic, metal or another material that a physician inserts into or through a body

---

71   *Lock Asylum Committee (1836–1842)* (The Library, Royal College of Surgeons of England, London), MS0022/2/1/4.
72   Siena, *Venereal Disease Hospitals and the Urban Poor: London's Foul Wards 1600–1800*, 235–241.

passageway to diagnose or treat a condition – and "then instruments used to keep the urinary tract from closing due to ulceration".[73]

In this chapter, the notion of fallen woman and the issue of female sexuality have been discussed; I have tried to demonstrate how the medical discourse surrounding middle-class ideology was behind ideas about prostitution and venereal disease, and how throughout the eighteenth and nineteenth centuries treatments have evolved and patients were the concern of both moral reformers and medical authorities. In the forthcoming chapters, all these ideas will be analysed in the light of the functioning and running of two unique institutions in the history of medicine and philanthropy in Great Britain, the London Lock Hospital and Asylum. Gender issues will be the object of my concern, especially in the cure and reform of female patients and in the different stages of the Hospital and Asylum throughout the nineteenth century.

---

73   Siena, *Venereal Disease Hospitals and the Urban Poor: London's Foul Wards 1600–1800*, 246.

CHAPTER 3

Female Patients and the Lock Hospital Regulations throughout the Nineteenth Century

The beginning of the nineteenth century brought with it the discourse of social medicine which was based on the surveillance and regulation of the poor to avoid immorality and the spread of contagion and disease to the decent population. The idea that financial expenditure should be checked was behind the debate over state intervention and public funding. This idea was shared by both Tories and Whigs in Parliament. Issues connected with the health of the people were the province of local authorities and voluntary initiatives. Therefore, the moral and medical concepts of health and disease focused increasingly on the habits and moral atmosphere of the working poor, and hospitals and similar institutions began to apply the new technologies of social disciplining based on the mental and physical regulation of inmates. Illness and corruption were associated with the lower classes, and were considered as natural in them.[1] As far as sexually transmitted diseases were concerned, the struggle between classes and faiths provided the context for changing attitudes at the turn of the eighteenth century. Sexual control and social restraint together with love of God and respect for non-religious authorities were increasingly propagandised as characterising the middle classes. Diseases such as cholera or syphilis began to be seen as the punishment of sinners, and things such as drunkenness, dirtiness or any other kind of uncontrolled behaviour were regarded as causes of infection and contamination. Thus, both the working poor and the aristocracy were stereotyped as improvident and ungovernable, and were categorised as deviant from middle-class normality. In this context, language was a powerful

[1] Frank Mort, *Dangerous Sexualities: Medico-Moral Politics in England since 1830*, 2nd ed. (Routledge: London and New York, 2000), 13–19.

tool for identifying those who did not comply with moral and social rules; words like rebels, culprits, or sinners were appropriated by the discourse of medicine and religion to identify those who had contracted venereal disease. The aim was to propagate an image of sexuality as something dangerous and to provoke fear of "the dreadful distemper" among the population.² As a result, voluntary institutions and, in particular, lock hospitals, were conceived for providing physical cure for venereal disease and to promote cleanliness, good habits and decent sexual behaviour during the time of convalescence, favouring reflection upon past sins as the result of vice. All these ideas can be found reflected in the regulations that the London Lock Hospital implemented throughout the nineteenth century, although an evolution can be appreciated between the Laws of 1814, 1840 and 1890. The latter had also many aspects in common with the rules governing other institutions of seclusion like prisons, workhouses or asylums, which were governed by the same principles of surveillance and control of the social deviants.

The regulations that the London Lock established in the nineteenth century for patients and staff reflect the way in which these types of institution tried to control and contain two of the most dreaded elements in Victorian society: prostitutes and fallen women. The London Lock Hospital also followed the principles that governed voluntary institutions described in the previous chapter, and the middle-class conceptualisations of respectable and unrespectable behaviour prevailed throughout the organisation and running of this philanthropic endeavour. These norms reproduced the double-standard of morality which established separate realms of action for men and women as described in Chapter 2. The aim was to keep order and decent behaviour in the patients and to teach them to act according to middle-class standards. For this, the religious and medical discourses formed an alliance to support social attitudes concerning gender and class. The first set of laws regulating patients and staff at the London Lock Hospital in the nineteenth century appeared in 1814 and was printed by Meredith and Son, Mount Street, Lambeth, by

2   Richard Davenport-Hines, *Sex, Death and Punishment: Attitudes to Sex and Sexuality in Britain since the Renaissance* (London: Fontana Press, 1991), 158–161.

Order of the Annual General Court held on 21st April of that year. Thus, the first section of *An Abstract of the Rules and Orders for the Government of the Lock Hospital near Hyde-Park Corner, Instituted July 4, 1746, for the Relief of Venereal Patients Only* is devoted to the Governing Body, which consisted of a Patron, a President, twelve Vice-Presidents, two Treasurers and a number of Governors. Governors – both gentlemen and ladies are explicitly mentioned – had to contribute yearly with a minimum of five guineas, becoming Subscribers, or to give a donation of 50 pounds or more, becoming Benefactors, that is, Governors for life.[3] The same regulations regarding the funding of the hospital and the prerogatives of Governors thereby can be found in the *Laws of the London Lock Hospital and Asylum of 1840* that were published in a little book with blue covers by Chapman Printer, Star Street, Paddington. The Institution was at the time under the patronage of HRH the Duke of Cambridge, with the Duke of Sutherland as its President.[4] The version that this manuscript contains is the revision of June 1848, with the Asylum Regulations at the end. The book contains notes on the margins written in the 1860s with corrections, suppressions and additions to these rules, which suggest that these norms were dynamic and changing, according to the necessities of the Institution.

Governors had the right to attend at all Weekly, Quarterly and Special Boards and to speak and vote on all questions. According to the significance of their contribution, they could recommend a number of in-patients and out-patients. The Weekly Board was held every Thursday at twelve o'clock, where patients were admitted following the recommendation of letters brought by Governors, although urgent cases without letters could be admitted by the Surgeon; also patients were discharged after reports by the physicians and surgeons. This Board had powers "to appoint, and confirm,

3 *An Abstract of the Rules and Orders for the Government of the Lock Hospital near Hyde-Park Corner, Instituted July 4, 1746, for the Relief of Venereal Patients Only, By Order of the Annual General Court held April 21, 1814* (The Library, Royal College of Surgeons of England, London), MS/0022/5/3.
4 Members of the Royal Family and the aristocracy were patrons and presidents of the Institution – as they were, of course, of a wide range of hospitals and other charitable institutions.

and suspend, and remove the house-surgeon, the apothecary, the collector, the secretary, the matron, porter, surgery-man, nurses, and all other servants", and this gives us an idea of the importance of the role of this body, which could also regulate and give directions concerning the duties of all the officers and servants in the Hospital. Similarly, each month a deputation was appointed by the Board "to inspect the wards and receive any complaints from the patients".[5] This was one of the very few ways in which the patients' voices could be heard; however, there are no surviving records in connection with this practice. The Weekly Board had also to examine and order the payment of all the bills, and to purchase the things the Hospital needed, ordering repairs and alterations when they were deemed necessary, but financial matters were in the hands of the Treasurers, the Trustees and the Collector. Treasurers and Trustees were elected for life, although subject to suspension or removal. The first would receive and give receipts for the money the Hospital obtained and would keep an account of all the transactions, safeguarding the keys of the poor-boxes and controlling donations from the middle-class congregation during services in the Lock Chapel to contribute to the maintenance of the Institution.[6] Treasurers would put the Hospital money in a bank account and keep insurance in their names as well, whereas Trustees would invest the funds of the Hospital, following directions of the different Board meetings. Collectors were recommended by Treasurers and were in charge of collecting the money from subscriptions and benefactions, although they appeared and disappeared at different stages in the history of the Hospital, working on commission.[7]

As has already been mentioned in Chapter 1, the Chaplain was an essential figure at the London Lock, not only for his role in the religious instruction

---

5   *Laws of the London Lock Hospital and Asylum, Revised (1840), 1848* (The Library, Royal College of Surgeons of England, London), MS0022/5/2.
6   Poor-boxes were kept at the Chapel, and both the Treasurer and the Chaplain had the keys to them; at service, they circulated through the congregation who put their donations in them to contribute to the running of the Hospital and Asylum.
7   *An Abstract of the Rules and Orders for the Government of the Lock Hospital near Hyde-Park Corner, Instituted July 4, 1746, for the Relief of Venereal Patients Only, By Order of the Annual General Court held April 21, 1814*, MS/0022/5/3.

Female Patients and the Lock Hospital Regulations   61

and reformation of patients, but also for the fundamental source of income that sermons and services at the Chapel represented for the Institution. There is no description concerning the duties of the Chaplain in the *Abstract* of 1814; however, in the *Laws* of 1840, he is presented as a member of the Church of England who had to be in full orders. He was appointed by the Trustees of the Lock Chapel. Rev. James Gibson and Rev. Thomas Garnier were chaplains at the time these rules were approved and then revised.[8] The Chaplain had to provide religious services at the Institution and carry out the instruction of patients, visiting them in the wards once a week "to perform all such religious offices, either by consolation or exhortation, or administration of the sacrament of the Lord's Supper". He had also to recommend books for patients to read so that their moral reformation was implemented, and to inform the Weekly Board of "all abuses and irregularities" that he witnessed.[9] However, the Chaplain's most important role was the salvation of sinners like prostitutes and fallen women. Although forgiveness was emphasised, punishment remained essential and deviant women had to repent their past life and ask forgiveness for their sins. The focus of rescue work became redemption and the reclamation of the sinner's soul, and this idea would promote the concept of the prostitute as a victim of social injustice so that "the parable of the lost sheep was used constantly as a comparison between rescue work, prostitution and religion".[10] There were very slight differences in the *Laws* of 1890 concerning the role of the Chaplain: he or his deputy had to perform the same duties with patients as far as religious services and instruction was concerned, recommending books and visiting the wards "at least once a week". What was new was the possibility of patients receiving that indoctrination by "ministers of legally certified places of worship", that

---

8   Rev. James Gibson was appointed Chaplain in 1811 and resigned in 1818; he was appointed Chaplain again in 1832 till 1847 when Rev. Thomas Garnier succeeded him. *Correspondence and Plates* (The Library, Royal College of Surgeons of England, London), MS0022/6/3.
9   *Laws of the London Lock Hospital and Asylum, Revised (1840), 1848*, MS0022/5/2.
10 Paula Bartley, *Prostitution: Prevention and Reform in England, 1860–1914* (London and New York: Routledge, 2000), 31–33.

is, of other denominations different from the Church of England, as long as notice was given by the Matron to the Chaplain.[11]

In harmony with the middle-class concept of the home, the London Lock Hospital and Asylum were based on a regime that reproduced the organisation of a respectable household with two crucial officers who represented the idea of the paterfamilias and decent wifely respectability: the Secretary and the Matron. They represented male and female authority and were the models that many, both male and female, patients were supposed to follow. One of them had always to be in the Institution at times when the other was absent. The Secretary was responsible for all the minutes of the different Boards and Committees, and was in charge of all the official documents of the Institution such as letters, accounts, books and deeds. He also had to keep a list of all the Governors, Subscribers and Benefactors, and to enter new or amended rules in the book for the *Laws of the London Lock Hospital and Asylum*. The Secretary had a salary and lived in the premises. He was in charge of all the businesses related to the male patients and the male servants and nurses in the male wards of the hospital. This meant that he had to inspect and visit these wards at least once a day, and he had to attend the Chapel of the Hospital every Sunday, together with the patients, nurses and servants in the male wards. According to these *Laws*, "He shall be master of the household, and as such, shall, in conjunction with the matron, be responsible to the Weekly Board for the order and good government of the household in every respect".[12] In all these senses, he represented masculine power according to the principles of 19th century England as a kind of household head for the Hospital. From these rules concerning the Secretary, who was in charge of the male wards and male officers and servants, and from those concerning the Matron who was in charge of the female, we can observe that the principle of segregation was kept at the London Lock Hospital. This was the common practice by the middle of the century, keeping male and

---

11   *Laws of the London Lock Hospital and Asylum (Rescue Home) 1890* (The Library, Royal College of Surgeons of England, London), MS0022/5/11. This last version of the London Lock regulations was printed by Burt and Sons, 58, Porchester Road, Bayswater, W., London.
12   *Laws of the London Lock Hospital and Asylum, Revised (1840), 1848*, MS0022/5/2.

female patients apart. The religious principles of the Church of England governed the rules and routines of this Institution. The Secretary's duties and prerogatives did not differ much in the *Laws* of 1814, 1840 and 1890, except for the role that the Ladies' Committee played in the management of the Female Hospital at the end of the century.

The Matron was another outstanding figure in the London Lock. Together with the Secretary, she had to reside in the House, and was paid a salary. According to the 1840 regulations, she had to fulfil a series of requirements: she had to be single and without family, to be between thirty and forty-five at the time of her election and would cease to be matron at the age of sixty-five. She had to be a respectable woman of good reputation and a member of the Church of England, reproducing then the middle-class moral standards. Like the Secretary, she had to visit the female wards once a day and read aloud the rules to nurses and patients at least once a week; all the nurses and female servants were under her supervision, and she was also in charge of the Asylum inmates. She represented the female authority that was sanctioned in all Victorian discourses, limiting her functions to the private sphere and keeping her appropriate gender roles. She had to have an irreproachable behaviour and be an example for the female inmates and, like the Secretary, she had to attend services in the Chapel every Sunday together with all female servants and patients. The Matron had power to dismiss any nurses and female servants at her own discretion as well, communicating irregularities or improprieties to the Secretary and the Weekly Board. She was also in whole charge and control of the Asylum and its inmates.[13] In the regulations of 1814, the Matron is also responsible for all the household goods, furniture and so on and was obliged to keep an inventory of them. Similarly, she was in charge of keeping an account of all the meat, bread and daily provisions for the Hospital meals, controlling the different diets for patients.[14] For example, in 1821, the diet for patients was as follows:

13 *Laws of the London Lock Hospital and Asylum, Revised (1840), 1848*, MS0022/5/2.
14 *An Abstract of the Rules and Orders for the Government of the Lock Hospital near Hyde-Park Corner, Instituted July 4, 1746, for the Relief of Venereal Patients Only, By Order of the Annual General Court held April 21*, 1814, MS/0022/5/3.

	Full	Half	Low
Breakfast	1 pt. gruel	1 pt. gruel	1 pt. gruel
Dinner	¾ lb meat	½ lb meat 4 days	1 pt. broth
	½ loaf of bread	1 pt. broth 3 days	⅙ loaf bread
	1 pt. beer	⅙ loaf bread	½ lb potatoes
		¾ lb potatoes	
Supper	1 pt. gruel	1 pt. gruel	1 pt. gruel[15]

These diets were elaborated according to the Surgeons' instructions by the Matron, and were very similar to others that could be found in various institutions for the poor like prisons, workhouses, general hospitals, penitentiaries, asylums, schools, etc. The Visitors' Book is mentioned and there are some of them which have survived in the London Lock archives; these books were very common for voluntary institutions and in them the impressions and opinions of visitors and subscribers were kept. They were under the custody of the Matron, and they were another instance of the exertion of middle-class control over these places of confinement and over the behaviour of the working poor. Among the Matron's duties was also to keep all patients' belongings, money, clothes, and so on, and to be in possession of the keys to all Hospital doors. She was to make sure that "the street be always locked up at eight in the evening, and not open till seven in the morning, from *Michaelmas* to *Lady-Day*; and be locked up at ten in the evening, and not open till six in the morning, from *Lady-Day* to *Michaelmas*, unless otherwise ordered by the Weekly Committee".[16] (Italics in original) It can be inferred from these regulations

---

15   *Correspondence and Plates* (The Library, Royal College of Surgeons of England, London), MS0022/6/3.

16   *An Abstract of the Rules and Orders for the Government of the Lock Hospital near Hyde-Park Corner, Instituted July 4, 1746, for the Relief of Venereal Patients Only, By Order of the Annual General Court held April 21,* 1814, MS/0022/5/3.
     Michaelmas was the feast of Saint Michael the Archangel celebrated in the Western Christian calendar on 29 September. Because it falls near the equinox, it is associated in the northern hemisphere with the beginning of Autumn and the shortening of days; Lady Day is the traditional name of the Feast of the Annunciation of

that not only patients but also nurses and other servants were unable to leave the Institution without the Matron's permission, and that in the nineteenth century the London Lock was really "locked".

However, during the Victorian period as a whole, there was a change in the roles and qualifications of the hospital matrons. Until the 1870s, their functions had been associated with efficient housekeeping, supervising all domestic arrangements of the institution concerning laundry, cooking and cleaning. Matrons had not been trained nurses until the last decades of the nineteenth century when they were recruited more from women and fully trained nurses. They were also called "Lady Superintendents" by this time and began to be something more than housekeepers. They were also in charge of the nurses' training at this stage and their new powers and education sometimes brought them into conflict with medical authorities. Altogether, being a hospital matron became an important career path for women at the end of the Victorian era.[17] By the 1890s, matrons at the London Lock had to be between the ages of thirty and fifty at the time of their appointment, and were in the first place accountable to the Ladies' Committee. The Ladies' Committee was responsible for the Female Hospital and the Asylum, and consisted of the Chaplain and a selected number of ladies who supervised the domestic arrangements under the approval of the Board. They met once in a month and arranged that one of them visited the Matron regularly, being a consulting body for her, providing advice, cooperation and support.[18]

The medical officers at the London Lock had rules to follow too. According to the 1840 regulations, the London Lock Hospital had a Consulting Physician and a Physician appointed but, as had happened in the past, they did not get involved very much in the affairs of the Institution.

---

the Blessed Virgin that takes place on 25 March in the Western liturgical year of English-speaking countries. Michaelmas and Lady-Day are two of the four traditional English quarter days, being Midsummer Day (24 June) and Christmas Day (25 December) the other two.

17 Michelle Higgs, *Life in the Victorian Hospital* (Stroud, Gloucestershire: The History Press, 2009), 124–127.

18 *Laws of the London Lock Hospital and Asylum (Rescue Home) 1890*, MS0022/5/11.

We must bear in mind that venereal disease was considered by physicians as a complaint whose treatment represented a kind of inferior practice. Therefore, their role at the London Lock was basically to give prestige to the Institution, devoting their efforts to more prestigious medical establishments. By contrast, surgical appointments were much more contested and there was a hierarchy among the various posts. The new acquisitions were designated Assistant Surgeons to be later promoted to Surgeons after their predecessors were raised to the condition of Consulting Surgeons. The latter do not appear in the manuscript of the *Laws* and were not expected to attend patients, although they used to participate in Governors' matters.[19] All patients had to be seen by a Surgeon or Assistant Surgeon twice a week, or even oftener in more urgent or serious cases, except out-patients who were attended less frequently. The surgeons were appointed for life, and one of them would examine all the people applying to be admitted into the Hospital every Thursday and would give a report to the Weekly Board of those who should be accepted as patients. Surgeons had the power to order admission of urgent cases that then had to be sanctioned by the same Weekly Board and could take pupils for surgical practice in the Hospital. During the 19th century, pupils were medical students who paid a sum of money to established surgeons or physicians to be instructed at various London hospitals so that they could start a practice of their own. In the case of the London Lock, a Pupil had to pay to the Surgeon who monitored him an entrance fee of six guineas for six months, or twelve guineas for twelve months, becoming eligible for the position of House Surgeon.[20] In the rules of 1814, the figure of the House Pupil is mentioned as a kind of superintendent for the rest of the Pupils, being in charge of the dressing and undressing of patients. He lived and boarded in the House, and some of his functions were later transferred to the Apothecary, whose main duties consisted "in carefully preparing and dispensing the medicines prescribed by the Medical Officers, in having charge of the drugs and other matters

---

19 David Innes Williams, *The London Lock: A Charitable Hospital for Venereal Disease, 1746–1952* (London and New York: Royal Society of Medicine Press Ltd., 1995), 53.
20 *Laws of the London Lock Hospital and Asylum, Revised (1840), 1848*, MS0022/5/2.

relating to the shop; and that he keep an account therof, and permit no waste or improper use of them".[21]

The House Surgeon was designated among those Pupils who had finished their apprenticeship in London or the provinces and wanted a practice in the capital that would allow him to meet senior members of the profession.[22] The House Surgeon at the London Lock was appointed for 12 months – and later for six – and had to report to the Board the number of vacant beds, of patients admitted during the week and of those about to be discharged in that period. He had to pay an amount of sixty pounds to the existing Surgeons to continue his training, attending them during their visits to the wards.[23] In the regulations of 1890, the House-Surgeon is mentioned in relation to the Harrow Road Hospital and Out-patient Department. As in the previous rules, he had to see that the patients were properly dressed and that the physicians and surgeons' directions were complied with. House-Surgeons were the only ones allowed to administer anaesthetics at this stage of medical practice, with the exception of a properly qualified person. The House-Surgeon had to visit the wards in the mornings and evenings every day and assist the Surgeon in the attendance of Out-patients, and would not allow medical men or others to visit the female wards. The House-Surgeon might have to attend women at the Asylum, and had to issue certificates that women who were to be removed from the Kinnaird Ward to the Asylum were fit for service and free from venereal complaints. He had also to keep a record of patients in the Ward Case Book with their date of discharge, the reason for treatment (whether gonorrhoea, primary or secondary syphilis) and also the Patient's Diet Card or Bed Ticket. Unfortunately, none of these documents have survived.[24]

21 *An Abstract of the Rules and Orders for the Government of the Lock Hospital near Hyde-Park Corner, Instituted July 4, 1746, for the Relief of Venereal Patients Only, By Order of the Annual General Court held April 21,* 1814, MS/0022/5/3.
22 Innes Williams, *The London Lock: A Charitable Hospital for Venereal Disease, 1746–1952,* 53.
23 *Laws of the London Lock Hospital and Asylum, Revised (1840),* 1848, MS0022/5/2.
24 *Laws of the London Lock Hospital and Asylum (Rescue Home) 1890,* MS0022/5/11.

Nurses were the most controversial figures in the Hospital system of the nineteenth century. The public discourse on nursing in the mid- to late-Victorian period covered issues of gender and class, together with aspects of hospital organisation and the care of patients. By the mid-nineteenth century, these issues were related to questions of health and sanitation, as we shall see.[25] In the first half of the century, most nurses in voluntary hospitals had been drawn from the same class as that of the patients and their role had been quite limited. Working conditions, salary and accommodation were not encouraging at all, and there was no training system.[26] Although hospitals made efforts to hire respectable women, the fact that words like "that they do not presume to take any reward, fee, or gratuity, of any Patient, or their friends, before admission, during their residence in the Hospital, or after his or her discharge from thence, under pain of being discharged by the next Weekly Committee" can be read as referring to the Nurses is quite revealing as to the moral and social character imputed to these women.[27] The rules also established that in the event of the death of a Patient, Nurses had to return all his or her belongings to the Matron and they were advised not to show any partiality to any individual patient. It is clear that they were susceptible to bribery. Among their duties by 1814 were keeping the wards clean and giving patients the appropriate medicines. They were to check patients' behaviour, forestalling the mixing of inmates in the male and female wards, and taking care that they were in bed by seven in winter and eight in summer.[28] Another interesting feature of the nursing profession in the early Victorian period was the existence of Anglican sisterhoods more or less modelled on Roman Catholic organisations. One of the most outstanding of these institutions was St. John's House that was founded in 1848 to train nurses to look after the sick poor in hospitals and homes. There were two

---

25   Arlene Young, "'Entirely a Woman's Question'?: Class, Gender, and the Victorian Nurse", *Journal of Victorian Culture* 13, 1 (2008): 18.
26   Higgs, *Life in the Victorian Hospital*, 128.
27   *An Abstract of the Rules and Orders for the Government of the Lock Hospital near Hyde-Park Corner, Instituted July 4, 1746, for the Relief of Venereal Patients Only, By Order of the Annual General Court held April 21, 1814*, MS/0022/5/3.
28   Ibid., MS/0022/5/3.

kinds of trainees: lady probationers and ordinary trainees. The first were of a superior class, paid a fee and worked on a voluntary basis; the latter were of a lower social rank and received in return board and wages.[29] The orders negotiated contracts with hospitals, but no allusion can be found to sisters in any of the London lock archives.

Things began to change by the 1850s after the Crimea War broke out and Florence Nightingale became involved in nursing as a profession. The demand for nurses to attend wounded soldiers brought with it the necessity of having better-qualified ladies to work in medical institutions. Nightingale herself opened a training school at St. Thomas's Hospital, where women were required to possess deep morality and spiritual devotion, together with a basic education and the hardiness of a working-class girl. Like matrons, nurses had to be single or widows without any family dependants, and resided in a nurses' home. During the period of training they were called probationers and after finishing it were known as sisters. Nightingale nurses had to sign for six years, and after the first year of training, they could be sent where they were needed. Probationers could be evaluated with a grading system that included "excellent", "good", "moderate", "imperfect" or "o" in the following fields of expertise: dressings, applying leeches, enemas, management of trusses and uterine appliances, rubbing, dealing with helpless patients, bandaging, making beds, waiting on operations, cooking for the sick, keeping wards fresh, cleanliness of utensils, management of convalescents, and observation of the sick.[30] Some of these activities show the kind of treatments and care patients received by nineteenth century standards; others may seem ridiculous if compared to contemporary nursing; and many were clearly associated with womanly tasks. But after 1867, Nightingale decided to recruit better-educated women to be trained for nurses; these ladylike probationers became known as special probationers and paid for their board and lodging to become superintendents, that is, matrons.[31]

29 Young, "'Entirely a Woman's Question'?: Class, Gender, and the Victorian Nurse", 23.
30 Higgs, *Life in the Victorian Hospital*, 129.
31 Ibid., 128–129.

Following the regulations of 1840, the London Lock Hospital hired nurses who were appointed by the Matron, and there were also Head Nurses and Night Nurses who had to obey the orders of the Secretary and the Matron. They had to be between thirty and forty-five at the time of their appointment, and had to be literate. This last requisite is very significant and gives evidence of the rising standards that began to be applied to these women in the second half of the nineteenth century and of the problems that the Hospital had probably had with nurses' behaviour in the past. Their obligations and routines did not change much in comparison with the 1814 rules: they could not leave the Hospital without the Matron's written permission, had to go to service in the Chapel every Sunday, and had to inform the Head Nurse of the death of a patient. Head Nurses had to observe that patients followed the directions of medical officers, and inform Night Nurses of the orders that had to be observed during the night.[32] A large supply of young women was always needed, as many left the profession because of marriage, which was one reason for resignations together with leaving one post for a better one in another hospital.

Another important issue was the decline in the number of male nurses in hospitals. Nursing was becoming a women's profession towards the end of the Victorian era and was associated with the women's sphere. However, male nurses did exist, and the public seem to have accepted them throughout the period. They were especially suitable for tasks considered inappropriate for women such as shaving and catheterising men, and they were part of the staff in most military hospitals and mental asylums.[33] It can be presumed that they were also quite indispensable in venereal facilities with male wards and male outpatients; in fact, a Surgery-man or man's Nurse is mentioned in the London Lock regulations of 1840, and in the rules of 1890 it can be read: "The male Nurse at Dean Street shall be appointed by the Board".[34]

---

32   *Laws of the London Lock Hospital and Asylum, Revised (1840), 1848*, MS0022/5/2.
33   Young, "'Entirely a Woman's Question'?: Class, Gender, and the Victorian Nurse", 36–37.
34   *Laws of the London Lock Hospital and Asylum (Rescue Home) 1890*, MS0022/5/11.

Similarly, and as nursing became gradually a more professionalised ladylike activity, conflicts between doctors and sisters began to arise and hospital management changed from the old system to the new one where nurses were not trained in the wards as a kind of informal apprenticeship any more, and boards of directors started to invite nursing sisterhoods and training programmes to their hospitals. Superintendents were hired and nurses rotated from ward to ward every three months to gain experience in all types of nursing care, with relations of power and resistance beginning to be the common feature of the relations among the medical staff.[35] However, these changes cannot have affected the Lock Hospital much, as it was a specialist hospital and segregation was practised between the wards and between the male and female servants.

As far as patients' rules were concerned, they had their precedents in the London hospitals of the eighteenth century with foul wards like St. Bartholomew's or St. Thomas's, and the London Lock itself. Hospitals had endorsed corporal punishment of foul patients in the seventeenth century, but there are no records of these activities being continued in the eighteenth. However, there were other ways of controlling transgressive inmates like withdrawing food rations for minor offences or immediate discharge for more serious ones. Other features of eighteenth century hospitals were the strict control of patients' eating and sleeping, preventing patients from leaving the premises, mandatory religious instruction, and the prohibition of things like swearing, theft, fighting and drinking. Although these regulations had been designed to disempower patients and avoid acts of resistance, many found ways to exert agency through refractory behaviour expressed by disobeying hospital rules, causing disruption in the wards by annoying nurses and other patients, committing thefts or staying out of the hospital during the night. Another way of subverting power was inciting other patients to act against the norms. Many escaped the institutions without finishing their treatment when symptoms began to abate because they could not

---

35 Young, "'Entirely a Woman's Question'?: Class, Gender, and the Victorian Nurse", 26–27.

stand the strict discipline and the harsh treatment.[36] Similar rules can be found in the London Lock for 1754, although they were less strict than in other hospitals of the time: patients were not "locked", that is, they could leave the hospital, provided that they were granted permission. In contrast with other hospitals where inmates had to partake in housekeeping activities, venereal patients did not have to perform any labour at the London Lock in the eighteenth century;[37] they were urged to behave in a decent and quiet way, avoiding gambling and quarrelling and following the instructions of the medical staff, but nothing was mentioned about religious instruction. By contrast, workhouse rules were even harder, with an established routine and inmates kept within the confines of the institution; physical punishment was quite common, as well as isolation in case of disobedience.

Generally speaking, both out-patients and in-patients had to follow hospital rules: the more serious their symptoms, the more thorough the rules. Out-patients were also expected to bring letters of recommendation from subscribers, and if they did not return regularly on the stated dates, they forfeited the right to treatment and were discharged. Sometimes they had to provide phials or galipots for their medicines.[38] An example of a letter of recommendation is this one from the Lock Hospital in the eighteenth century:

> Gentlemen
> To the Governors of the Lock Hospital I desire you will admit into your Hospital the Bearer _____ of the Parish of _____ (if h____ Case entitles h____ to the Charity) being well assur'd _____ is a proper Object, and am Your Humble Servant.[39]

---

36 Kevin Siena, *Venereal Disease Hospitals and the Urban Poor: London's Foul Wards 1600–1800* (Rochester: University of Rochester Press, 2004), 122–123, 130.
37 Ibid., 188–189, 247.
38 Higgs, *Life in the Victorian Hospital*, 51.
39 Siena, *Venereal Disease Hospitals and the Urban Poor: London's Foul Wards 1600–1800*, 228.

Thus, in-patients for voluntary hospitals had to be in possession of an "admission ticket" once a letter of recommendation had been provided, and had to present themselves on the day and at the time stated in the ticket. The ticket used to list the personal items that patients had to bring with them. This practice varied from hospital to hospital.[40] In the case of the London Lock, the rules of 1814 stated that "every Patient do bring with him or her, two shirts, or shifts, and two pairs of stockings".[41] As has been already stated, having a governor's nomination did not always guarantee a bed in a voluntary hospital, and when there was no room for more patients, these were put in a waiting-list. But they seem never to have been refused. In most hospitals, patients would stay for a maximum of six weeks under the same ticket, which was a long period of time compared to contemporary standards. Tickets could be renewed by surgeons or physicians at their own discretion and according to the patients' situations, but many of them were sent to a convalescent home because they needed more time for their complete recuperation.[42]

A copy of the rules was always displayed in the wards and published in many annual reports. According to the 1814 *Rules*, London Lock Patients had "to take the Medicines prescribed by the Physicians or Surgeons, and administered by the Nurse; and behave quietly and decently while they were under cure"; they could not move out of their wards and must be in bed by seven in winter and eight in summer.[43] These rules also obliged patients to help nurses in the running and keeping of the wards, as long as this physical activity was not, in the surgeons' opinion, detrimental for their recovery. This meant a significant change in comparison with the Hospital rules in the eighteenth century. In particular, women were expected to perform certain chores such as maintenance of wards, needlework and laundry work; these

---

40 Higgs, *Life in the Victorian Hospital*, 55.
41 *An Abstract of the Rules and Orders for the Government of the Lock Hospital near Hyde-Park Corner, Instituted July 4, 1746, for the Relief of Venereal Patients Only, By Order of the Annual General Court held April 21, 1814*, MS/0022/5/3.
42 Higgs, *Life in the Victorian Hospital*, 58.
43 *An Abstract of the Rules and Orders for the Government of the Lock Hospital near Hyde-Park Corner, Instituted July 4, 1746, for the Relief of Venereal Patients Only, By Order of the Annual General Court held April 21, 1814*, MS/0022/5/3.

tasks were very often quite hard, and many of the inmates were unwilling to perform them. Men were in charge of repairs and other activities which were associated with masculinity and physical strength.[44] Differences of sex and class were reinforced in these hospitals, and the penalty for transgressing these regulations was expulsion, with the impossibility of being readmitted into the London Lock. Most patients in the London Lock Hospital were therefore working-class, and men and women from the superior classes who suffered from venereal disease went to private doctors to obtain treatment, as has already been mentioned. The women patients were considered deviant, promiscuous and riotous and the perception of their lives of sin was biased by middle-class standards; only some married women and mothers were regarded as decent by the authorities running the Institution. Not only homes and penitentiaries but also lock hospitals taught women submissiveness and patriarchal values, accepting the supervision of the medical officer and then the matron, who was set as an example of proper feminine behaviour. Again, women were taught middle-class social and moral values, and were trained to return to the private sphere as domestic servants.[45] The working classes were identified as "filthy", "unruly" and "disordered" and naturally predisposed to immorality by the middle classes, and their life conditions and physical constitutions were considered determinant for their moral degeneration. During the nineteenth century, they represented the fear of the "Other", and the process of genderisation was evident in describing morally deviant men as "cowardly", "small", "emasculated", "solitary" or "with a want of a manliness of feeling", while morally deviant women were described as "vulgar", "insubordinate", "indelicate", "aggressive", "obstinate" or with "unwomanly and offensive habits". These bodily inscriptions were the outward manifestation of transgressive interiorities which, in the case of women, signified lack of respectability through the appearance of the "Other". Working-class women's bodies were thus seen as the sites of difference and monstrous identities being the vessels of promiscuity and

---

44 Judith R. Walkowitz, *Prostitution and Victorian Society: Women, Class and the State* (Cambridge: Cambridge University Press, 1991), 221.
45 Ibid., 222–223.

contagion. As a consequence, moral pathologies were the production of particular social discourses produced in particular social contexts, with an inferiorisation of working-class cultural traits expressed through physical differences and ways of living which differed from bourgeois decency and propriety. Infectious bodies should therefore be confined and removed from their community and fellow citizens to avoid the propagation of vice, and this was the spirit behind the London Lock Hospital and other institutions for the seclusion and reform of the morally deviant.[46]

This is the reason why in the regulations of 1814, activities usually associated with the working classes like gambling, drinking, swearing or rioting were forbidden for the patients, being an example of the prejudices that the bourgeoisie had against the lower orders who frequently categorised them as the "undeserving poor". In the same fashion, Patients could not receive any food or drink from Visitors or people outside the Hospital, but had to follow the House Diet. Similarly, bribes were forbidden so that Patients could not "give to any Nurse, Officer or Servant of this Hospital, any money, gratuity, fee, or reward, for any services done or to be done".[47] Similar rules for patients can be found in the *Laws* of 1840, but there was a slight difference concerning their admission: instead of being put onto waiting lists, urgent cases would be accepted and the others would become out-patients until they could be admitted into the House. In the same vein, they had to behave with "civility, decency and sobriety", and if they disobeyed the norms they could be expelled and would not be readmitted.[48]

At this time, many important changes were taking place at the London Lock, and the moral results of the Female Patients for the year 1847 totalled

46 Heidi Rimke, "Constituting Transgressive Interiorities: Nineteenth-Century Psychiatric Readings of Morally Mad Bodies", in *Violence and the Body: Race, Gender and the State*, ed. Arturo J. Aldama (Bloomington, Indiana: Indiana University Press, 2003), 250–255, 259.
47 *An Abstract of the Rules and Orders for the Government of the Lock Hospital near Hyde-Park Corner, Instituted July 4, 1746, for the Relief of Venereal Patients Only, By Order of the Annual General Court held April 21,* 1814, MS/0022/5/3.
48 *Laws of the London Lock Hospital and Asylum, Revised (1840), 1848*, London, MS0022/5/2.

as follows: of a total of 148 women admitted into the Lock Hospital, 23 were married, 24 were placed in asylums, 4 were discharged for bad conduct, 6 absconded, 12 were restored to friends, 71 had gone and nothing was known about their whereabouts, and 8 remained in the Hospital.[49] These figures reflect all that has been said above: many of these women were rebellious and could not stand the strict regime, like those who fled or the ones who were discharged for misbehaviour; they also show the number of married women under treatment. This strongly suggests that male adultery was quite common among the lower classes, but this figure was similar to the number of women who were sent to the Asylum and thus regarded as suitable for further reform. Some were restored to friends or remained in the Hospital to continue their treatment, but the number of women whose destination was unknown after discharge is really disturbing. It can be presumed that some of them lived in lodgings or worse, that they had nowhere to go and had to resort to the streets again. In any case, the success of the Hospital in its moral and sanitary function is more than questionable.

In the 1840s, the lease for the Grosvenor Place location was expiring and the Trustees of the London Lock addressed the owner of the property, the Marquis of Westminster, who expressed his intention of not renewing the ownership of the land for the purposes of the Institution. He, nonetheless, manifested his intention of maintaining the lease for another year. A Building Committee was established in 1839 and it held its first public meeting on the 8th of June of that year at the Thatched House Tavern, St. James Street, with the Duke of Cambridge in the chair, as patron. A new location was found for the Hospital, Asylum and Chapel in Harrow Road, and different appeals were made separately for the different buildings. Several meetings were held at the Thatched House Tavern, and these accelerated the project's realisation. The foundation stone was laid on 29th of May 1841; the Asylum would be incorporated in the same building as the Hospital. Separate appeals were further made for the completion of the Hospital and Asylum, and the building of the Chapel for 6,000 and 4,000 pounds respectively in 1842.

---

49 *Cuttings Album* (The Library, Royal College of Surgeons of England, London), MS0022/11.

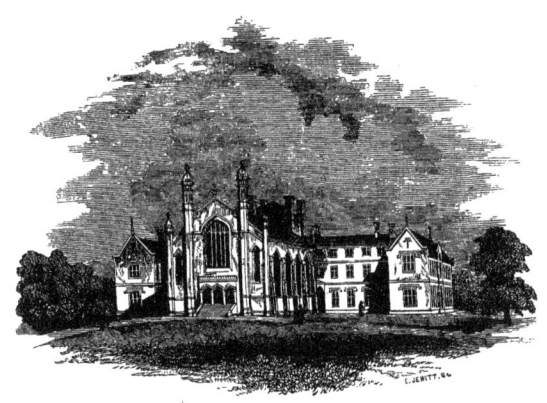

APPEAL for £6000.

TO COMPLETE THE ASYLUM FOR PENITENT FEMALES,

IN CONNEXION WITH THE

LOCK HOSPITAL, WESTBOURNE GREEN,

Now only capable of receiving 20 Inmates.

AND TO FINISH THE ERECTION OF THE HOSPITAL ITSELF.

CHAIRMAN OF SUB-COMMITTEE:
H. R. H. THE DUKE OF CAMBRIDGE.

Committee:

VISCOUNT MORPETH, M. P.	GEORGE BURNAND, ESQ.
LORD KINNAIRD.	REV. T. GARNIER.
ROBERT BENSON, ESQ.	REV. E. HOLLOND.
WILLIAM BENSON, ESQ.	JOHN LONG, ESQ.
GEORGE BIRD, ESQ.	MAJOR MACFARLANE.

Honorary Secretary:
THE HON. A. KINNAIRD.

AMONG the admirable purposes to which it was proposed to appropriate the Public Order Memorial Fund, not the least important and desirable was that of affording assistance to established Institutions, restricted for want of funds. Few existing charities have on this ground a greater claim on the liberality of the Public, than the *Lock Asylum.*

Above one hundred and fifty degraded daughters of the poor, for the most part of a very tender age, pass through the adjoining Hospital in the course of the year. The greater proportion of these having been faithfully instructed during their residence in the Wards, express the most earnest desire to be saved from their life of shame. But whither can they go? Exasperated relatives spurn them from their doors. Virtuous families refuse to employ or shelter them. Even the Asylum established for this very object, in

Front Cover Appeal for 6,000 pounds to complete the Asylum for Female Penitents, Cuttings Album, the Library, Royal College of Surgeons of England, MS0022/11.

On 18th of June 1842 the new building was officially opened and the inaugurating sermon was preached by the Chaplain who pronounced the following words:

> O God, from whom all holy desires, all good counsels and all just works do proceed, we thank thee for having put it into the hearts of thy servants to found this refuge for the sick and the penitent. Knowing that without Thee nothing is strong, nothing is holy, we humbly beseech thee so to bless this undertaking that many unhappy sufferers may receive a bodily cure and that the diseases of their souls may be healed by the wholesome medicines of Thy holy words, to the glory of Thy name, through Jesus Christ our Lord, Amen.[50]

These words maintain the idea of the London Lock as an Institution that can deal with both patients and penitents, providing them with physical treatment and religious instruction, so that both the body and soul of the deviant can be cured. New appeals were made again to finish the Asylum and Chapel in 1843, and the new Chapel was finally inaugurated on the 30th of May 1847.

The 1890 rules contain only a few regulations for the patients with very few changes to those of 1840. For example, patients were not readmitted when discharged for irregularity at this stage either, with the exception of a workhouse order when there was a fresh attack of venereal disease. Also, out-patients could not remain under treatment for a period longer than eighteen months, unless they had the Board's approval. What was new is the inclusion in the Secretary's copy of a separate document with the Hospital rules, which reads as follows:

1. At 6 a.m. patient to rise. Trip beds, turn mattresses and open windows at the direction of the nurse and leave beds to air. Wash and dress in lavatories.
2. Make beds and tidy wards before breakfast.
3. 7–7.45. Morning prayers and breakfast.

---

50 *Patients Records, Correspondence and Plates, An Account of the Lock Hospital, from notes taken from the Minute Books* (The Library, Royal College of Surgeons of England, London), MS0022/6/3.

4. 10 a.m. Ward, lavatories and bathroom to be in perfect order.
5. Morning hours to be occupied in needlework, writing letters, reading or attending in surgery if required.
6. 12 noon. Dinner.
7. 2 p.m. The afternoon and evening to be spent in reading and needlework except when services are being held in the wards.
8. 4 p.m. Tea.
9. 6.30 p.m. Supper, followed by prayers.
10. 8 p.m. All patients to be in bed and lights lowered. No talking allowed afterwards.
11. Bad language and disorderly conduct or talking over wrong-doing are also strictly forbidden.
12. All letters for patients will be opened by the Matron, and such as are objectionable, will not be given.
13. The nurses are authorised to report to the Matron any breaking of the rules or disobedience to those in authority.

Note. Patients are invited to co-operate in the carrying out of these rules which are framed for the general welfare and comfort of the inmates.

BY ORDER.[51]

These thirteen rules encompass all the principles that were followed concerning the routine and behaviour of patients at the Lock Hospital: order and cleanliness in the wards and for the inmates' bodies; religious instruction with prayers and services; work and daily routines so that patients were not idle at any time; and the surveillance of patients through their correspondence and even their conversations. The same control was exerted over visitors, with strict visiting hours for family and friends, and the numbers of visitors per patient limited.

In conclusion, the various London Lock regulations throughout the nineteenth century do not show much difference with other voluntary

---

51 *Rules for Patients in Hospital* (The Library, Royal College of Surgeons of England, London), MS0022/5/3.

institutions for confinement during the period. The aim behind these rules was to control and contain the behaviour of working-class patients who represented a threat to middle-class order, and to subjugate their identities, especially in the case of women, to eliminate all the traits of working-class life. The presence of the principles of the Anglican Church is more than evident, and the attempt at reforming the destitute poor with venereal disease is part of a philanthropic project which found many instances of resistance in the challenging conduct of some of the patients or their leaving the Institution as soon as the symptoms of the illness had disappeared, or even before. Thus, the London Lock Hospital is a classic example of England's architecture of containment of the working classes, particularly the morally deviant.

CHAPTER 4

The London Lock Hospital and the Contagious Diseases Acts: Reports and Accounts

The years before the passing of the Contagious Diseases Acts were a period of change both for the Hospital and society, and a premonition of the turmoil and social uproar of the forthcoming decades. The sentimentalism that pervaded the first decades of the nineteenth century concerning the figure of the prostitute and fallen woman gave way to other considerations. The notion that a woman's sexual fall should be attributed to masculine depravity began to lose preponderance, although the idea of seduction was ever present in the discourses of Magdalenism that impregnated the rescue work of the middle decades of the century.[1] However, connections between health and disease, morality and immorality were further established and the power relations between men and women concerning their sexuality were similarly upheld by the medical and religious discourses that became essential by the middle of the century. The functioning of Institutions like the London Lock was an example of the Foucauldian idea of power as both "regulatory and productive" in terms of "bodies, pleasures and desires", that is, in terms of knowledge.[2]

With the passing of the Public Health Act of 1848 and the creation of the General Board of Health, a turn in the medical and moral policies concerning the regulation of sexuality gathered pace. Immorality was identified with working-class life and with uncontrollable behaviour that could spread to the rest of the "decent" remainder of the population. In the 1840s,

---

[1] Michael Mason, *The Making of Victorian Sexual Attitudes* (Oxford and New York: Oxford University Press, 1995a), 86–87.
[2] Frank Mort, *Dangerous Sexualities: Medico-Moral Politics in England since 1830*, 2nd ed. (Routledge: London and New York, 2000), 2–5.

sexual depravity was identified with urban squalor and in particular with the living conditions of the poor: the lack of sanitation, personal hygiene, and overcrowding of working-class dwellings. Because of the latter, incest became one major source of moral preoccupation for the middle classes that also identified the notions of dirt and illness with urban disorder. These ideas were reinforced by Evangelicalism and other religious currents which resorted to a language of animal carnality to describe the sexual immorality of the working poor. In this sense, working-class men were seen as brutalised and lacking any kind of morality, whereas working-class women were viewed as immoral pollutants, and these ideas presided over the power-knowledge relations that affected the middle- and the lower-classes in the middle years of the century.[3]

In contrast with this, the middle-class woman was supposed to be respectable and to have a reputation which was based on the lack of sexual desire, and the middle-class man was supposed to be able to exert control over his sexual instincts and to avoid excess.[4] The sexual identity of the bourgeoisie was constructed over the themes of "health, hygiene, procreation and inheritance".[5] As a result, moderation was advised for men and regular habits for wives and children to avoid the dangers of sexual excess. Nevertheless, the reality was that the late age of marriage and the social constrictions that circumscribed the lives of the middle classes influenced the sexual behaviour of men who had to find release for their sexual needs with mistresses and prostitutes, and there were opinions for and against these practices within the medical profession. The same controversy dominated the question of masturbation, although the medical stance concerning this matter was more unanimous.[6] Masturbation was widely reprobated and seen as a dangerous activity, not only in children and adolescents, but also in young adults, and involuntary nocturnal emissions were also considered

---

3   Mort, *Dangerous Sexualities: Medico-Moral Politics in England since 1830*, 29–31, 37.
4   Lesley A. Hall, *Sex, Gender, and Social Change in Britain since 1880*, 2nd ed. (London: Palgrave Macmillan, 2013), 16–17.
5   Mort, *Dangerous Sexualities: Medico-Moral Politics in England since 1830*, 33.
6   Michael Mason, *The Making of Victorian Sexuality* (Oxford and New York: Oxford University Press, 1995b), 183–184.

as a threat to middle-class morality. Doctors believed that the consequences of both activities were very alarming as they provoked spermatorrhoea in men and the waste of semen that was lost to the continuity of the English breed and to fruitful intercourse within marriage. Many devices and remedies were applied to avoid erection and in a punitive way in most cases, and some of them were designed by quack doctors who proliferated in a business which was outlawed from serious medical practice. In the case of women, the focus of fear was on the clitoris, and some doctors believed that many of the female maladies that threatened the physical and moral health of the female sex were related to self-abuse.[7]

Masturbation was closely connected with pornography, which was a flourishing trade that reflected Victorian sexual anxieties. Pornography had been traditionally associated with radicalism and free thought in the working classes, but by the middle of the nineteenth century it became a middle-class business. The production of pornographic books was transformed into an expensive commercial activity with a very limited market that only the literate and the rich could afford.[8] Thus obscenity became one of the most important objects of concern in metropolitan culture as many London shop-windows displayed pornographic images that offended the sexual prudery of the respectable classes. Holywell Street, just off the Strand, became the most visible place where most pornographic materials were exhibited and could be purchased, which became the focus of persecution under the Obscene Publications Act of 1857. This piece of legislation had as its main aim to control the visibility of obscene materials and avoid their circulation, and gave powers to the police to destroy anything they judged subversively erotic.[9]

In this new atmosphere, the London Lock Hospital saw a period of movement concerning the physical location of its installations which

---

[7] Hall, *Sex, Gender, and Social Change in Britain since 1880*, 26–27.

[8] Roy Porter and Lesley Hall, *The Facts of Life: The Creation of Sexual Knowledge in Britain, 1650–1950* (New Haven and London: Yale University Press, 1995), 152–153.

[9] Lynda Nead, "From Alleys to Courts: Obscenity and the Mapping of Mid-Victorian London", *Sexual Geographies, New Formations: A Journal of Culture/Theory/Politics* 37 (1999): 33–41.

affected male and female patients with an increasing number of people seeking relief from a physical ailment which was spreading alarmingly throughout the metropolis and the rest of the country: syphilis. There were two main objects of concern for the Governors of the Institution in the 1850s: the creation of an out-patient and male Department in some central part of London and the completion of the existing building which had moved to Harrow Road, Westbourne Green after the expiry of the lease in Grosvenor Place. This last change meant that the London Lock had broken its links with St. George's Hospital and had created new ones with St. Mary's Hospital as a teaching hospital and as far as the medical staff was concerned.[10] The new connection between the London Lock and St. Mary's Hospital would last for over a hundred years.

There were several reasons for the formation of an Out-patient Department and a male hospital in a different location. The new site for the Hospital and Asylum signified larger installations for patients and penitents but at the same time the distance between the Westbourne Green area and central London was considerable. The painful character of the disease and the destitution of those seeking for cure of venereal complaints rendered it almost impossible to cover the distance either on foot or paying any type of conveyance. Also, the need to stop the advance of the illness at its early stages and to benefit from the free advice and medicines that the Charity provided made it imperative to have a building in the centre of the metropolis. Other arguments were put forward, like London being the only large city in Europe to lack appropriate hospital accommodation for male and female venereal patients, or the need to stop the spread of an affliction that could lead to the moral deterioration of the race and be transmitted to successive generations.[11] In November 1851, a special appeal was therefore authorised by the Court of Governors to give permission to the Weekly Board to find suitable premises for the Male and Out-Patient

---

10   David Innes Williams, *The London Lock: A Charitable Hospital for Venereal Disease, 1746–1952* (London and New York: Royal Society of Medicine Press Ltd., 1995), 61.
11   *Extract from the Annual Report, 1st January, 1855, Cuttings Album* (The Library, Royal College of Surgeons of England, London), MS0022/11.

Department. The 1850s saw years of economic prosperity after the death of the previous Treasurer, Charles Hoare, and the appointment of his successor, Arthur Kinnaird, who also served as Chairman for many years and had a very relevant role in the negotiations for the central London dependencies and the running of the Hospital under the Contagious Diseases Acts. Income and expenditure were kept balanced at this time, and the debts of the Hospital had been paid by July 1858; the Chapel was also flourishing and a paid apothecary was appointed in 1854.[12] The new building for the male patients and the Out-patient Department was finally located at 91, Dean Street – close to Soho Square – and accommodated 60 beds for male patients in a small ward on the first floor with large out-patient facilities on the ground floor. New medical staff was needed to attend male out-patients four days a week and the female ones just one day a week, so that the two sexes did not get mixed.[13]

There were various reasons for enlarging the building in Harrow Road. The most important one was the possibility of having many more rooms and increasing the number of beds for female patients, which would give Governors the possibility of remedying the situation of many more suffering sinners. However, as the century progressed there was an increasing tendency to classify different individuals who were the object of charity and, in particular, the types of women received by the Institution. They needed to be categorised in Foucauldian terms according to their degree of deviancy.[14] In this sense, a distinction was to be made between the "profligate", the "degraded" and the "immoral" from innocent married women and children. The increased number of beds would even allow for the admission of private patients of "superior station" who would require the service of the Surgeons at the London Lock. To all this was added the idea

12 *Patients Records, Correspondence and Plates, An Account of the Lock Hospital, from notes taken from the Minute Books* (The Library, Royal College of Surgeons of England, London), MS0022/6/3.
13 Innes Williams, *The London Lock: A Charitable Hospital for Venereal Disease, 1746–1952*, 73–74.
14 Michel Foucault, *The History of Sexuality: Volume I, An Introduction*, trans. Robert Hurley (London: Penguin, 1990), 17–35.

of having a convalescent ward for the Lock Asylum as an intermediate step for women between leaving the Hospital and entering the Asylum, where potential penitents could receive the care and advice of the Matrons and Chaplain. In this way, the sincerity of penitents' resolutions to atone for their past lives and start new ones in the path of morality and virtue could be tested.[15] Similarly, in 1859, the idea of transforming the London Lock into a Clinical School with the physician, surgeons and assistant surgeons teaching medical students under the regulations of the Weekly Board was also contemplated[16]

The *Reports of the Lock Hospital, Asylum and Chapel* for the 1850s were written by the Rev. W.H. Hind, the Assistant Chaplain during these years, who compiled very useful information about the patients regarding their birthplace, origin, education, religious denomination, social condition, moral condition and their destination after leaving the Hospital. The analysis of all these aspects will allow us to establish an accurate picture of the types of individuals seeking help on the premises. The first element that attracts the reader's attention is the significant increase in the number of sufferers admitted by the Hospital in these years. Apart from the fact that the number of beds had risen substantially after the completion of the West Wing in 1849, the policy of the Hospital had also changed and cases were accepted not only at the suggestion of Governors who took in "every case requiring immediate medical attention, without any recommendation whatever but their own need", but also by the decision of surgeons.[17] Thus, the number of patients admitted in 1855 was 211, 455 were admitted in 1856 – 210 male and 235 female –, 428 in 1857 – 211 male and 217 female –, 387 in 1858 – 186 male and 201 female –, and 397 in 1859 – 218 male and 179 female –, as the *Annual Reports* for 1856, 1857, 1858, 1859 and 1860 show, in contrast with the smaller numbers of previous years. These figures show a rough gender-balance, but they do not

15 *Extract from the Annual Report, 1st January, 1855, Cuttings Album*, MS0022/11.
16 *Patients Records, Correspondence and Plates, An Account of the Lock Hospital, from notes taken from the Minute Books*, MS0022/6/3.
17 *Report of the Lock Hospital, Asylum, and Chapel, 1853* (The Library, Royal College of Surgeons of England, London), MS0022/4/2.

give names. The patients presented all kinds of ailments and conditions. At this stage both sexes were still treated at Westbourne Green, and most patients were suffering from "secondary or tertiary syphilis, chancroid, complicated gonorrhoea or venereal warts",[18] with a significant number of male out-patients despite the existing distance between the city centre and the Hospital, whose male premises had not yet moved to Harrow Road. Treatment remained mainly unchanged, and, although the speculum began to be used for diagnosis in women by Samuel Lane, who was appointed Assistant Surgeon to the Lock in 1851, acute gonorrhoea was still treated with balsam of copaiba and culebs by mouth or irrigations of the urethra, strictures with bougies, and syphilis with mercury, sometimes using fumigation. The only innovation was the use of potassium iodide. At the same time some operations were undertaken by surgeons with the use of chloroform.[19]

The statistical information that the *Reports* provide between 1856 and 1860 is most useful to understand the ways in which the London Lock Hospital and Asylum operated in the middle of the nineteenth century. An overwhelming majority of patients came from London and its vicinity, followed by a considerable number of cases from the provinces, and only a few from abroad. During these years the London parishes sent their parishioners affected by venereal complaints, and contributed to their treatment at the London Lock. Among these parishes, those more frequently mentioned by Hind were Marylebone, Kensington, Paddington, Lambeth, St. Pancras, Lower Chelsea, St. James and St. Margaret, Westminster, St. Georges, Hanover Square, and Hammersmith, that is, those located in central London. The sole peripheral parish was Hammersmith.[20] The fact that a few of the inmates of the Hospital came from continental Europe and even the colonies is quite significant, even though their precise number cannot be determined because they are mixed with those from the provinces.

18 Innes Williams, *The London Lock: A Charitable Hospital for Venereal Disease, 1746–1952*, 68.
19 Ibid., 71–72.
20 *Reports of the Lock Hospital, Asylum, and Chapel, 1856, 1857, 1858, 1859, 1860* (The Library, Royal College of Surgeons of England, London), MS0022/4/2.

However, these numbers can be rather telling as to the presence of foreign prostitutes and to the possibility of the existence of an international trade in prostitution in England and particularly in London, both from and to the continent, despite the tendency of social and cultural historians to dismiss the possibility of white slavery, especially in connection with the Stead affair which will be discussed in a succeeding chapter.

Regarding the birthplace of patients, here again most inmates of the Hospital had been born in London and the Provinces, and the counties which appear in the *Reports* are Kent, Middlesex, Essex, Bucks, Surrey and Wilts, that is, near London in most cases. This meant that the Hospital served these areas besides the metropolis, and some of the patients are also referred to as foreigners.[21] As a consequence, in the *Report* for 1858, claims are made to "the benevolent support of the wealthy landowners, the merchants and manufacturers of the Provinces, as well as the nobility, gentry, and merchants of London".[22]

Even more interesting is the question of age. With the exception of the *Report* for 1856, where the majority of inmates oscillated between 18 and 21 years of age, and the one for 1860 which does not include that information, the rest of these accounts include the ages of patients differentiated by their gender, as shown in the following table:

Ages Male/Female	13–16		16–18		18–21		21–26		26–30		+30	
1857	1	5	8	51	62	82	66	73	34	13	39	11
1858	1	9	10	53	45	79	79	54	32	12	44	9
1859	2	4	14	45	45	77	55	55	33	8	33	10

These numbers give us a clear idea of the situation regarding the age of sexual initiation for women who entered the Hospital. With the exception of an infant in the *Report* for 1858, and of one male and two females under

---

21 Ibid., MS0022/4/2.
22 *Report of the Lock Hospital, Asylum, and Chapel, 1858* (The Library, Royal College of Surgeons of England, London), MS0022/4/2.

13 for the *Report* for 1859, female patients start to be recorded when they are 13, which means that they began to have sexual intercourse – maybe after rape – between the ages of 13 and 16, entered prostitution and contracted venereal disease about two years later. This explains the difference in numbers from the male patients, whose presence in the Hospital was more common at later ages. Similarly, these figures allow us to establish a connection between the situation of these young girls and the issue of the age of consent and the debates it provoked in the last decades of the nineteenth century. They also show that women remained in prostitution till their late twenties and that their clients resorted to them until their thirties. These figures are coincident with the ones given by Tait for Edinburgh Lock Hospital or by the Chief Constable of York and the York Penitentiary Society returns for the 1840s.[23]

The other questions touched upon in the *Reports* for these years give us quite an accurate notion of the character of most male and female patients in the Hospital. According to Hind, the two most important characteristics of these inmates were their lack of morality and their ignorance. A significant number of them could not read or write, but there was a wide spectrum of patients who ranged between the capacity to read and write well, the capacity to do it tolerably, the capacity to do it indifferently, and those who could read only. It seems that books were taken to the wards for those literate patients who wanted to make use of them during their stay in hospital. However, the most outstanding feature of patients was their lack of "morals", especially in the case of females. In most *Reports* for the 1850s the majority of women patients were prostitutes – some of them had been living in concubinage –, and a considerable number had been either "privately wanton" or the victims of seduction. The notion of "prostitute" became quite ample in the middle decade of the century, encompassing a "constellation of women's behaviour which moral reformers found objectionable or threatening".[24]

---

23 Frances Finnegan, *Poverty and Prostitution: A Study of Victorian Prostitutes in York* (Cambridge: Cambridge University Press, 1979), 76, 81.
24 Linda Mahood, *The Magdalenes: Prostitution in the Nineteenth Century* (London and New York: Routledge, 1990), 68–69.

Therefore, prostitutes became socially constructed categories; they were the object of debate and were subjected to control. However, the causes of women's fall were varied, including economic need, seduction, and the attractions of a life of pleasures and riches. Nonetheless, Hind saw the influence of peers and a defective moral training were especially influential. There were a few exceptions of married women and widows who sometimes were of an unblemished character, and this is the reason why he recommends the division of the classes inside the Hospital, following the trend of those years in rescue work.[25] By the middle of the century prostitutes were abundant in London, and there were many institutions which aimed to redeem them, paying more attention to their moral degradation than to the diseases they suffered from and spread.[26] Special allusion is made to intemperance which affected male patients and led them to their evil courses, especially in places of working-class recreation:

> The remark made in last Report [sic] as regards the connexion between the indulgence of intoxicating liquors, and the sin which fills your Hospital, is fully borne out in the cases of the male patients received during the past year. The half-conscious votary of intemperance, as he reels from the gin-palace, is seized upon by a painted siren, and borne off by her to a den of infamy and ruin. To the gin-palace, dancing saloon and theatre, a large proportion of the gross vice in our country is fairly chargeable.[27]

Prostitutes had an extra source of income taking their clients to the brothel or public house and making them drink, the same as brothel-keepers implemented their earnings by renting their rooms to prostitutes and by obtaining the returns of their clients drinking alcohol on their premises. Also, thefts and fights were very common, as was noted in Chapter 2. However, most clients were widely said to be inebriate before soliciting the prostitutes' services.[28] Later in the century, temperance reformers like

---

25 *Report of the Lock Hospital, Asylum, and Chapel 1857* (The Library, Royal College of Surgeons of England, London), MS0022/4/2.
26 Innes Williams, *The London Lock: A Charitable Hospital for Venereal Disease, 1746–1952*, 61.
27 *Report of the Lock Hospital, Asylum, and Chapel 1858,* MS0022/4/2.
28 Finnegan, *Poverty and Prostitution: A Study of Victorian Prostitutes in York*, 108, 125.

William Logan in his book *The Great Social Evil* (1871) identified drink as one of the main causes of prostitution. In this sense, Rev. Hind mentions in the 1857 *Report*, the necessity of creating young men's Associations "founded on a truly religious basis, and affording both rational recreation and useful instruction" to distract men from the lure of alcohol and evil women. This link will be discussed later in the book.[29]

The social condition of both male and female patients was indicative of their family background and occupations, as well as their religious activity and their destination on leaving the Hospital. The fact that the 1856 *Report* mentions that some of the Patients had been dismissed for improper conduct, had left surreptitiously or had demanded their discharge, may well reveal that many of them belonged to the lower working class or that they could not bear the strict discipline and the religious instruction they were subject to. Of those who had been discharged cured, some had returned home or to their friends; others had entered or resumed service, but also there were others who had returned to their old ways.[30] In some of the other *Reports*, we are informed that some of the inmates entered other reformatory institutions or the workhouses they had come from. This information is also revealing: many patients of the Hospital had been sent by London workhouses which did not have venereal facilities for the destitute. The majority of patients were single, but among both male and female inmates were married men and women as well as widows and widowers. Regarding their occupation, the majority of women had been in service or other useful occupation, but there were quite a few who had never had any useful activity. The most common occupations among male patients were handicraftsmen, tradesmen and labourers; sometimes servants and clerks are mentioned as male patients' professions.[31] We can therefore infer that most people looking for relief from venereal complaints were of the lower social orders.

29 *Report of the Lock Hospital, Asylum, and Chapel 1857*, MS0022/4/2.
30 *Report of the Lock Hospital, Asylum, and Chapel 1856* (The Library, Royal College of Surgeons of England, London), MS0022/4/2.
31 *Report of the Lock Hospital, Asylum, and Chapel 1857*, MS0022/4/2.

As has been stated before, religious instruction was very important in the daily routine of patients in the Lock Hospital. At this stage, most of them belonged to the Established Church, but there were some "Romanists" – Catholics – and a smaller number of Wesleyans, Independents, Baptists, Presbyterians, Lutherans, and even Jews and Plymouth Brethren, although in some cases a person's faith could not be ascertained or they had not been baptised. According to the 1857 *Report*, there were many inmates who were ignorant of the first principles of the doctrine of Christ, and, although many of the females were said to show contrition and repentance from their former lives, these feelings were not always lasting.[32] Despite the fact that the members of the medical profession and the clergy despised the ways of living of the working classes and their sexual depravity, they could offer them the promise of salvation and a better life enjoying health and longevity by winning the fight between flesh and spirit.[33] And this return to morality was officially offered by the London Lock Hospital and Asylum together with a physical cure.

The London Lock was hardly likely to remain unaffected by the broad shift of opinion towards regulating prostitution that led to the passing of the Contagious Diseases Acts in the 1860s. In those days, Dr. John Simon, who became first Medical Officer to the City of London in 1848, gave pre-eminence to the concept of preventive medicine based on a system of inspection and administration, and emphasising the importance of research. At this stage, the physical and moral cleanliness and health of its citizens became a fundamental principle for the state and its sanitary policy, displaying the Christian values and the humanitarian disposition of a civilised nation. From the 1850s onwards, there was also a tendency to specialisation and pathologisation of "deviant" individuals thanks to the emergence of environmentalism which influenced medicine, education, and rescue work.[34]

The Contagious Diseases Acts had several precedents which are worth investigating and analysing. Two of the most relevant ones are the venereal

---

32 Ibid., MS0022/4/2.
33 Mort, *Dangerous Sexualities: Medico-Moral Politics in England since 1830*, 32.
34 Ibid., 51–52, 58.

legislation in the British Empire and the proctorial system of regulation of prostitution in Oxford and Cambridge. In the first case, notions about sex and gender were intermingled with race; here, the work of Philippa Levine is particularly illuminating. According to her, between the 1850s and 1880s venereal legislation was passed and implemented in the British colonies around the world to put an end to metropolitan anxieties about the spread of sexually transmitted diseases among British soldiers, identifying female prostitutes as the main source of contagion. These regulations obliged these women to register and undergo periodical medical examination to detect venereal disease. The fact that the majority of the colonial population was male, military and unmarried favoured the representation of the soldier as a victim and of the colonial prostitutes as the origin of infection. Medical authorities endorsed the idea that the venereal poison was more potent and that sexual and moral laxity was greater in interracial settings than in Europe. Doctors in the colonies tended anyway to be more often in government service and to support racial hierarchy within the Empire, particularly after the shock of the Indian "Mutiny" in 1857.[35] Two issues were at stake: prevention and European manliness. There was no efficient treatment for venereal complaints at the beginning of the nineteenth century, and men in the British army could not be punished or policed, so the only way to control their sexuality was through the inspection and surveillance of prostitutes. Similarly, the fear of homosexuality and the idea that men had to give vent to their sexual instincts was behind this ideology of regulation in the colonies. It was essential to avoid violence, alcoholism, mutiny and desertion in soldiers.[36] Officer-patients would probably seek private advice which would certainly be more discreet and effective.

Throughout the Empire, it was physical contact between the English male coloniser and the colonised indigenous female that linked into an anyway increasingly virulent debate about race. Indigenous women's

---

35 Philippa Levine, *Prostitution, Race and Politics: Policing Venereal Disease in the British Empire* (Routledge: London and New York, 2003), 1–4.
36 Douglas M. Peers, "Soldiers, Surgeons and the Campaign to Combat Sexually Transmitted Disease in Colonial India, 1805–1860", *Medical History* 42, 2 (1998): 138, 147.

sexuality was assumed to be more relaxed and unrestrained than that of white women. In addition, the genital examination of colonial prostitutes could be better accepted than that of English or European prostitutes.[37] Racial inferiority was very much present in the colonial discourse about prostitution and was connected with assumptions about far-away societies' "oriental", "primitive" essence or cultural "depravity". British colonial imagination was plagued with fears about the threat to the superiority of the white, particularly the British, race and hence about the need to prevent racial mixing, which was equated with dilution of the British breed. Consequently, many of the ideas which encouraged the legislation to control promiscuity in the metropolis were inspired by the experience of regulation in the colonies.[38]

Similarly, the proctorial system in Oxford and Cambridge Universities was another antecedent for the Contagious Diseases Acts. The regulation of prostitution to protect scholars from both Universities was the result of a series of medieval privileges which survived into the first decades of the nineteenth century. In particular, Cambridge was a city divided into two communities, "town" and "gown". The first was composed of working-class people, many of whom were employed by the University; the second was of young men who formed an elite group isolated from female company and whose welfare was the responsibility of the University authorities.[39] Special university statutes allowed the Vice-Chancellor to examine suspected prostitutes in his Court, to register them and to subject them to a medical inspection if needed, which might lead to their incarceration if found venereally diseased. Public surveillance was guaranteed by the proctors and their agents – also called bulldogs – who patrolled the city at night to remove disorderly women from the streets.[40] After 1836, prostitution

---

37   Ibid., 149.
38   Levine, *Prostitution, Race and Politics: Policing Venereal Disease in the British Empire*, 6, 8.
39   Janet Oswald, "The Spinning House Girls: Cambridge University's Distinctive Policing of Prostitution, 1823–1894", *Urban History* 39, 3 (2012): 454.
40   Philip Howell, "A Private Contagious Diseases Act: Prostitution and Public Space in Victorian Cambridge", *Journal of Historical Geography* 26, 3 (2000): 378–379.

was also controlled by the borough police outside the University confines, and more specifically in the suburb of Barnwell where prostitutes served men of their own class and could be arrested under the vagrancy laws mainly as drunk and disorderly. Detained prostitutes were taken to the Spinning House, a refuge founded in the seventeenth century by Thomas Hobson where criminals and prostitutes were kept. They were made either to spin or to weave so as to contribute to their maintenance. By the 1820s, the House became the University prison for Cambridge streetwalkers. The building was located in St. Andrew's Street, very close to the Market Square where, along with the riverside area known as the Backs, most of the activity between prostitutes and students took place. The University of Oxford did not have a similar building, but suspected women were kept under the Clarendon building, and then sent to the city prison if they were convicted, with the Vice-Chancellor being obliged to pay a daily fee for them.[41] In Cambridge, there was much controversy among the non-University population in relation with the operations of the University concerning streetwalkers. This made University authorities cut the number of women being condemned and taken to the Spinning House from the mid-1850s. There was a slight increase in their numbers at the time of the application of the Contagious Diseases Acts in the rest of the country during the 1860s and 1870s, but by the 1880s the number of arrests significantly decreased again. This led to the closure and demolition of the Spinning House in 1901.[42]

As early as 1838, the idea of regulating prostitution had appeared on the agenda of Lord Melbourne who was then the Prime Minister. Coincidentally, Parent's text, *De la Prostitution dans la Ville de Paris* published in 1836, became the model for many English studies on prostitution that provided a European system of regulation that the United Kingdom could follow.[43] Regulation was timidly suggested for the first time in the

---

41 Janet Oswald, "The Spinning House Girls: Cambridge University's Distinctive Policing of Prostitution, 1823–1894", 459–460, 467.
42 Ibid., 469.
43 Mary Spongberg, *Feminising Venereal Disease: The Body of the Prostitute in Nineteenth Century Medical Discourse* (London: Macmillan, 1997), 37–38.

Lancet in 1843, and the question was explored in detail in a series of editorials three years later. After that, in 1850, *The Westminster Review* became clearly stronger in its advocacy of sanitary measures which would approach the issue against venereal disease; the emphasis was put on the fact that the disease spread from the guilty to the innocent.[44]

Another triggering event was the Crimean War (1854–1856) that led to the establishment of the Royal Commission on the Health of the Army of 1857 after the verification of the high incidence of venereal disease among the soldiers. The Report of this Commission advised ending the genital examination of military men because it was humiliating for them and at the same time ineffectual; to the same extent, it recommended improving their environmental conditions in the barracks and stopping the routine of their lives behind the lines. However, by then, there was a firm belief in the necessity of conducting a medical inspection of prostitutes as the source of contagion[45] The role of Florence Nightingale, who had famously been working as a nurse in the Crimea, was fundamental in the organisation of a Sanitary Commission in 1862 to deal with the issue of venereal disease in the military population. Her opinion was very relevant in the selection of its members, and she formulated many questions for the Committee. Nightingale was against the examination of prostitutes. In the same vein, Harriet Martineau published a series of letters in the *Daily News* in 1863 against the passing of venereal legislation. In the end, the Report of the Commission established that no system of regulation should be implemented following the European model, but it equally recommended the creation of voluntary lock hospitals and the improvement of sanitary conditions for soldiers who could be penalised for contracting venereal disease.[46]

---

44   E.M. Sigsworth, and T.J. Wyke, "A Study of Victorian Prostitution and Venereal Disease", in *Suffer and Be Still: Women in the Victorian Age*, ed. Martha Vicinus (Bloomington & London: Indiana University Press, 1973), 93–94.
45   Mary Wilson Carpenter, *Health, Medicine and Society in Victorian England* (Oxford: ABC Clio, 2010), 23, 84–85.
46   Judith R. Walkowitz, *Prostitution and Victorian Society: Women, Class and the State* (Cambridge: Cambridge University Press, 1991), 75.

Two prominent figures contributed greatly to the medical and social debate concerning prostitution and morality: William Acton, whose views on prostitution have already been discussed in Chapter 2, and W.R. Greg. Both men prepared the path for the acceptance of some type of regulation in the 1850s. Acton was an example of a medical authority in favour of the Acts and was committed to expansionist sanitary reform. He had worked among the poor of Islington and was medical consultant to the London Lock Hospital as a specialist in venerealogy. He was also witness to most Parliamentary enquiries on the issue of prostitution, and with his two books, *Prostitution* and *The Functions and Disorders of the Reproductive Organs*, both published in 1857, contributed to the primacy of medical statistics in the prevention and cure of illnesses. He asserted that male continence was necessary but that it could not be guaranteed because of the nature of man, and grew alarmed at the number of members of the lower ranks of the Armed Forces who had contracted syphilis or other sexually transmitted diseases. However, according to Acton, women lacked sexual desire. He found in biology the explanation for this behaviour: maternity and domesticity were women's essential instincts, and the sexual drives of the prostitute, the courtesan and the nymphomaniac were totally unnatural in his opinion. In this way, he established the polarisation between pure and impure women, which was behind the intellectual climate which endorsed the regulation of female behaviour in the 1850s and 1860s.[47] In the same fashion, Greg advocated the French system of regulation to be applied to British prostitutes when he talked about the "Great Social Evil" in his articles in the non-medical press, like the *Westminster Review*. For him, prostitution and venereal disease were one and the same thing. He thus ignored the role of men in the spread of the illness. Also, fears about the growing visibility of prostitutes and their degrading and troublesome behaviour contributed to the public awareness of the need for regulation.[48]

---

47 Mort, *Dangerous Sexualities: Medico-Moral Politics in England since 1830*, 60–61.
48 Mary Spongberg, *Feminising Venereal Disease: The Body of the Prostitute in Nineteenth Century Medical Discourse*, 56–57.

In the light of all these developments, the records of the Hospital House Committee between 1862 and 1872 kept in the Library at the Royal College of Surgeons of England are very significant about the way patients were treated and reacted and other aspects in the running of the Hospital. There was a Committee Board meeting where a Reverend was always present and where the Matron's opinion was very important; prayers were usually read at the beginning of the meeting. The minutes of the Board mention the existence of a Porter's Book which was laid before the Committee and a Ward Deputation Report was also read. An analysis of the minutes between October 7th 1862 and September 29th 1863 reveal substantial information during the days immediately before the passing of the first Contagious Diseases Act.[49] Throughout this year, we find information about women patients being admitted or discharged, about their ages and behaviour, about the reasons for their discharge, about their origin on admission and about their condition. Admittedly, their voices are never heard, but we can infer how some of them might have felt or thought through the interpretation, maybe not always accurate, of the details we obtain about them in the archives. Male patients are never mentioned, which implies that they were just admitted into the Hospital and discharged when cured or maybe at their own request; but their circumstances, names, ages or conduct seem to be of no relevance to the Board.

The names of female patients are often referred to, the same as their ages. These vary between 15 and 24 years; this fact confirms the tendency of the majority of women being admitted into the Hospital to be in their middle to late teens and early to middle twenties. The same trend has been observed in the *Reports* and *Accounts* of the Institution for previous years. The reasons why female patients were discharged from Hospital varied greatly, but are very telling as to their characters and ways of life. Some of them were released cured; some were sent home to their husbands or mothers; others were sent back to service, which was one of the main working-class occupations for women; some were sent to the Asylum; and

---

49 *Hospital House Committee, 1862–1872* (The Library, Royal College of Surgeons of England, London), MS0022/2/4/2.

also some deaths of female patients or their children did occasionally occur. There are also some examples in the archives of women who were released "at their own request", which probably meant that they could not bear the strict discipline, the religious and moral instruction or the hardness of the treatment. Nonetheless, misconduct was the reason for many discharges and, as stated before, this was attributed to the traits of working-class character by the middle- and upper-class benefactors of the Institution. For example, on October 7th 1862, Maria Furnell was discharged by the House Surgeon for insolence to the Matrons and quarrelling, and on February 10th 1863 the following can be read from the Ward Deputation Report in the minute of the Board meeting for that day: "Visited the wards, found that two of the patients Farrow and Varney have very much misconducted themselves, that they are incorrigible as to the use of bad language, and must be dealt with severely".[50] In the same vein, in the minute for December 16th 1862, one female patient, Dinah Neil, is reported to have "dirty habits", which were described as voluntary, and the "House Surgeon was requested to censure her publicly for same and if continued to dismiss her at once".[51] The allusion to these habits is again quite revealing: we can read that this woman either had a propensity to uncleanliness or to sexual misconduct.

Regarding admissions, female patients were accepted by the Board, but surgeons were allowed to accept urgent cases, as stated above. Only in a few instances did married women, such as Selena Kemp, enter with a child. Readmission was not very common, with the exception of a small number of cases, like women who were in the Asylum and were readmitted on account of ill health or pregnant women who had been sent to the workhouse in labour and then returned for treatment. An example was Louisa Jones, who was admitted again to the Hospital from Paddington Workhouse at the Board meeting of December 16th 1862. She had been sent to the workhouse on November the 27th in labour. This meant that pregnancies were not uncommon among female patients and that some babies began to be part of the daily life of the Hospital. At the same Board

50 *Hospital House Committee, 1862–1872*, MS0022/2/4/2.
51 Ibid., MS0022/2/4/2.

meeting it is even reported that another woman, Louisa Hastings, had been delivered of a child in the Hospital, probably because she did not know her possible date of delivery or because labour began sooner than expected. Finally, an operation on a female patient is referred to in one of the minutes, so this practice continued in the Hospital at this stage.[52]

We also know from the archives the places of origin of female patients during these years, as well as their places of destination when released. In particular, between 30th September 1862 and 29th September 1863, female inmates came from areas in London such as Woolwich, Hampstead Road, Fitzroy Square, Season Lane, Brompton Road, St. Pancras, Edgeware Road, Hanover Square, Lambeth, Harrow Road, Shrip Lane, Hammersmith, Drury Lane, Whitechapel, Walthanstow and St. Martin's Lane, and from localities like Windsor or Henley on Thames, despite their distance from the Hospital. Many of them came from workhouses of the neighbouring parishes like Mountcourt Workhouse, Paddington Workhouse, Islington Workhouse, Woolwich Union, or Hanover Square Workhouse. Similarly, many of the female patients were sent to the workhouse when released, and particularly to St. Pancras Workhouse, Kensington Workhouse, Eaton Square Workhouse, St. James's Workhouse, or Paddington Workhouse. Some of them were sent to homes or asylums like Portland Home, Harrington Asylum, St. Thomas's Home, or White Lion Home.[53] In other words, workhouses received female patients when discharged from the London Lock Hospital who did not have anywhere or family to go to and belonged to the parish; at the same time, London workhouse authorities sent women with venereal disease when they did not have lock wards or adequate facilities for treatment, and they had to pay a fee to the Hospital.

---

52 Operations to remove parts of the penis or the labia were also taking place as an invasive treatment of venereal disease in lock hospitals. However, their effectiveness was not clear, and the same happened with other measures taken such as the use of mercuric salts, potassium iodide purgatives, low diet, cauterisation of sores, etc. Probably, ablusions with soap and water, clean clothes and rest had more positive results. F.B. Smith, "The Contagious Diseases Acts Reconsidered", *The Society for the Social History of Medicine*, 3 (1990): 213.

53 *Hospital House Committee, 1862–1872*, MS0022/2/4/2.

With the New Poor Law of 1834, a network of workhouses was built throughout the country for each parish or for several small parishes which formed a Union; outdoor relief was abolished and women without support became the second largest population in workhouses after the elderly. Most of these women had been deserted by their husbands, were domestic servants between jobs, or widows, but a considerable proportion of them were what was known as "women of low character", that is, pregnant women or prostitutes who might be either in their early careers or hardened streetwalkers. Until 1839, unmarried mothers had to wear a yellow uniform and were secluded in the so-called "canary wards". Many gave birth to their children in the lying-in wards of these workhouse infirmaries, which were appalling in most cases.[54] In 1867, *The British Medical Journal* published two "Reports" about the Workhouse Infirmary of Clifton and the Workhouse and Infirmary of Northleach, which give as quite a detailed idea of how these Poor Law institutions worked at the time of the Contagious Diseases Acts. The Northleach Workhouse consisted of a Male Infirmary, a Women's Sick Ward, a Men's Fever Ward, a Women's Fever Ward that was used as a day and night nursery, and a Lying-in Ward as medical facilities; to these were added a Boys' School-room and a Girls' School-room, the Young Men's Dry Room, where most of the work like picking oakum was carried out by three very old men, the Men's and Women's Dormitories and the Able-Bodied Women's Ward, where seven women were contained, four of whom were illegitimate mothers and the other three were imbeciles. The condition of the building was quite good with the exception of the Men's and Women's Vagrant Wards that were close to the Chapel, because, according to the "Report",

> it should be borne in mind that workhouses are no longer penitentiaries for able-bodied idlers and lazy vagrants, but *homes* in which the declining years of most of our labouring population *must* be spent, and in which it is but simple justice that they should find no inconsiderable amount of home enjoyments. (Italics in original)[55]

54 Norman Longmate, *The Workhouse: A Social History* (Pimlico: London, 2003), 156–157.
55 "Report on the Northleach Workhouse and Infirmary", *The British Medical Journal*, November 16, 1867: 458–459.

In these words we find how the conception of the workhouse as a place of punishment for the idle members of the low orders and the poor was sometimes being transformed into an idea which contained the notion of providing the destitute old with a home where to spend their final days. However, the "Report" on the Clifton Workhouse Infirmary provides a more distressing description of life and conditions in these places of confinement with no supply of water on the upper floor of the building which was used by aged women. Also, the appalling state of the male itch and lock wards is underlined and the fact that these wards "were locked in at night without any means of communicating with a nurse if assistance was required" calls the reader's attention to how wretched and dismal were the lives of the people affected by venereal disease in these Infirmaries.[56] It is important to outline that from around 1860, most workhouses began to classify women in the female wards to separate the youngest, most innocent ones from the most depraved, following the tendency of those years. Despite the harsh rules, it was often quite difficult to keep discipline and order amongst these women whose conduct was not always desirable.[57] We can thus argue many similarities between various charity institutions in the nineteenth century as far as their inmates and organisation were concerned.

The Contagious Diseases Acts of 1864, 1866 and 1869 have been the object of debate and analysis both by contemporaries and social historians, and have become an emblematic example of the regulation of sexuality in the nineteenth century. However, their application and the changes brought about by them to the London Lock have never been explored and evaluated as far as their implications for the patients and the Institution were concerned. With them, the prostitute's body became the site of discrimination and sexual exploitation as well as the object of surveillance and control, and their physicality was inscribed with meanings of moral decay as vessels of disease.

---

56 "Report on the Workhouse Infirmary of Clifton", *The British Medical Journal*, November 9, 1867: 433.
57 Longmate, *The Workhouse: A Social History*, 59, 161.

And this was certainly the spirit behind the first Contagious Diseases Act of 1864, which was a provisional measure that was supposed to lapse, or be renewed, after three years. The title with which it was introduced in Parliament was "A Bill for the Prevention of Contagious Diseases at certain Naval and Military Stations", with a parenthetical note that read "not dealing with animals". In fact, the Act equated women with animals to a certain extent as we can infer from the language and legal connotations of the text, and succeeded some veterinary measures which were less problematic. The Bill was introduced to Parliament on 20 July by Sir Clarence Paget, Secretary to the Admiralty, and provoked very little debate; it had gone to Committee for amendments and the removal of some offensive clauses on 19 July, and on 21 July at two o'clock in the morning, with a House with only fifty men present, it was adopted. Finally, it obtained the royal assent on 29 July 1864.[58] A special body of policemen dressed in plain clothes was created from the Metropolitan police and was to work under the supervision of the Admiralty and the War Office independently from the local police: if a member of this force or a registered doctor believed that a woman could be a common prostitute – a term that was left undefined by this legislation –, he would inform a Justice of the Peace who would summon the woman to a certified hospital for medical examination. Women could submit voluntarily to inspection, but, if they refused, the magistrate could order to take them to hospital and examine them by force. The examination had to take place within a period of twenty-four hours and if a suspected prostitute was found venereally diseased, she could be detained in hospital for a period of up to three months. Hospitals had to be certified by an Inspector of the military, and for that they could not be more than fifty miles away from the intended district. Prostitutes who resisted medical inspection or did not comply with the hospital regulations were liable to punishment of one month's imprisonment for the first offence, and of two months for any subsequent one. Also, the Act provided magistrates with a clause that allowed them to prosecute keepers or owners of inns,

---

58 Spongberg, *Feminising Venereal Disease: The Body of the Prostitute in Nineteenth Century Medical Discourse*, 60, 63.

brothel-keepers, publicans, lodging-house owners, etc. that supported prostitutes and sentence them to a fine of up to 10 pounds or three months' imprisonment, with or without hard labour.[59] This first Act was passed as an exceptional step to protect soldiers and sailors from venereal complaints in eight garrison and dockyard towns in England – Aldershot, Chatham, Colchester, Plymouth/Devonport, Portsmouth, Sheerness, Shorncliffe and Woolwich – and three in Ireland – Cork, the Curragh and Queenstown.[60] Only half of the eight English districts implemented this piece of legislation, and the same probably happened in the Irish ones; to certify a hospital took quite a lot of requirements and the system needed time to start to work, acting in different ways in different places.[61]

In the case of the London Lock Hospital, with the application of the Contagious Diseases Acts of 1864, 1866 and 1869, Admiralty cases from Woolwich, the War Department and the Government were admitted and discharged from Hospital, and the number of patients

---

59   Philip Howell, *Geographies of Regulation: Policing Prostitution in Nineteenth-Century Britain and the Empire* (Cambridge: Cambridge University Press, 2009), 38–39; Paul Mc Hugh, *Prostitution and Victorian Social Reform* (London: Croom Helm, 2009), 37–38; E.M. Sigsworth and T.J. Wyke, "A Study of Victorian Prostitution and Venereal Disease" in *Suffer and Be Still: Women in the Victorian Age*, ed. Martha Vicinus (Bloomington & London: Indiana University Press, 1973), 94–95.

60   The case of Scotland, which had its own legislation, was different. The first time municipal authorities were given powers to close brothels and stop solicitation was with the Police Act of 1843, which had amendments in 1862 and 1866, but they did not work effectively till 1870 when McCall was made Chief Constable. The implementation of the law had very much to do with the support of the directors of the Lock Hospital and the Glasgow Magdalene Institution, combining a system of repression and reform. The Glasgow Police Act of 1866 "provided the municipal police and magistrates with extensive new powers to imprison or fine 'prostitutes' and brothel-keepers and to enter private property or any establishment suspected of harbouring 'prostitutes'". Mahood, *The Magdalenes: Prostitution in the Nineteenth Century*, 123–126. Therefore, both brothels and prostitutes became the object of surveillance and control in a way similar to that of the English Contagious Diseases Acts.

61   Howell, *Geographies of Regulation: Policing Prostitution in Nineteenth-Century Britain and the Empire*, 28, 43.

increased considerably, as the records state, although London itself was not included in the subjected districts.[62] As early as 1st December 1863, a letter was addressed to the Trustees of the Lock Hospital which read as follows:

> Gentlemen,
> I am commanded by my Lord Commissioners of the Admiralty to request that you will cause them to be informed whether it would be in their power to make an arrangement by which a certain number of Beds in the Female Wards of the Lock Hospital, London, may be placed at their disposal. If so, they would wish to know the actual costs for Beds.[63]

Mr. Kinnaird and Mr. Hare[64] took care of the matter, and at the meeting of the Weekly Board of 7th January 1864 it was agreed that the Governors would place a ward with 25 beds at the disposal of the Admiralty for a sum of 500 pounds per annum. The Lords of the Admiralty wanted the arrangement to be considered as an experiment to last for at least six months, and also decided to pay for the travelling expenses of women and their supply of linen and clothing as well as any charge for washing. Ten beds for women from the parish of Woolwich were also to be taken at a sum of 200 pounds per year, and 50 pounds a year were allocated for the Woolwich

---

62 *Hospital House Committee, 1862–1872*, MS0022/2/4/2.
63 *Patient Records, Correspondence and Plates*, "An Account of the Lock Hospital, from Notes Taken from the Minute Books", MS0022/6/3.
64 Arthur Kinnaird (1814–1887) served for many years at the London Lock, first as Treasurer and then as Chairman. He was the tenth Baron of Kinnaird and after holding an appointment in the foreign office at St. Petersburg, he became a partner in the banking firm of Ransom & Co. of Pall Mall East. He was a Liberal MP for Perth from 1837–1839, and from 1852 until 1878 when he succeeded his father as Baron Kinnaird. He was associated with many charitable organisations like Dr. Barnardo's Homes, London City Mission and the Aged Christians Society, besides the Lock Hospital. His wife was Mary Jane (1816–1888), daughter of William Henry Hoare. She was also a philanthropist and formed many benevolent institutions, including Y.W.C.A., the Zena Bible and the Medical Mission. Mr. Hare was the Secretary of the Institution at the time. Innes Williams, *The London Lock: A Charitable Hospital for Venereal Disease, 1746–1952*, 62.

Board of Health to pay for the travel expenses to send them from and to London, and for washing and the supply of linen for destitute cases.⁶⁵ The Admiralty and the War Office were going to make separate arrangements, but it was later agreed that the latter would supervise the whole process. The Army and the Navy appointed Inspectors to the London Lock Hospital (Mr. Leonard and Mr. Sloggett respectively), and medical examiners were recruited – a Dr. Stuart was appointed by the Army who examined patients from the local Board of Woolwich or the magistrates, and followed cases up in Westbourne Green.⁶⁶

In December 1864 a Committee of medical men was established, chaired by D.C. Skey, FRCS. Officially, it was to enquire into the pathology and treatment of venereal disease, but in fact it had as one of its main aims to determine the advisability of extending the Act. Its findings reinforced the idea of the female body as a site of infection and disease; as a consequence it should be policed in the same way as sewers or drains. So this legislation was seen as a sanitary measure to improve the health of the population, and the Committee was at the same time concerned about men with a weak "constitution" who were more likely to contract the disease. This can also be connected with the fears about homosexuality and the anxiety about deviant and unnatural sexual behaviours that began to appear in those years and were much more discussed in the final decades of the century. Almost all the witnesses that testified before the Committee were in favour of regulation and the extension of the existing Act. Only three of the sixty-three men who gave evidence had strong objections against the Act, and what was important is that their arguments were "entirely structured around notions of morality and immorality, cleanliness and pollution",⁶⁷ following the tendency of earlier years in the history of regulation. The most important principle behind the Committee's Report of

---

65 *Patient Records, Correspondence and Plates,* "An Account of the Lock Hospital, from Notes Taken from the Minute Books", MS0022/6/3.
66 Innes Williams, *The London Lock: A Charitable Hospital for Venereal Disease, 1746–1952,* 89.
67 Spongberg, *Feminising Venereal Disease: The Body of the Prostitute in Nineteenth Century Medical Discourse,* 70.

1866 was to remove the visible signs of venereal disease, that is, prostitutes. In this way, the identity of these women was clearly defined as "the other" and their banishment from decent society was a form of punishment for their immoral behaviour. The Committee eventually recommended that the periodical examination of prostitutes be made compulsory with the creation of a well-organised medical police. It also advised the extension of the Act to all naval and garrison towns, leaving the control of hospitals and police in the hands of the Government. But the Committee did not agree on the possibility of examination of males.[68]

The Contagious Diseases Act of 1866 was of unlimited duration and came to replace the previous after it had been repealed. Like its predecessor, it was introduced to Parliament by Sir Clarence Paget on 15th March 1866. It passed with little opposition and received the royal assent on 11th June 1866. The operations of the Act were extended only to Windsor – in fact, the Act would not be in full operation in all the subjected districts till 1870 –, and the Admiralty and War Office were given powers to appoint visiting surgeons and inspectors to registered hospitals or to add lock facilities in places where the system was in operation. When information was given on oath by the police that a woman was believed to be a common prostitute in the district, the magistrate could order her to go through periodical examination every two weeks for a period never exceeding a whole year. In most cases women volunteered and the power of magistrates was eroded as doctors were able to order the detention of women who had not submitted to the fortnightly examination. Again, if a woman was found venereally diseased she would be detained in hospital for up to six months, on the recommendation of a doctor; medical authorities could also transfer women from one hospital to another or to stop their examination altogether. Therefore, magistrates could only remove or include prostitutes in the register in reality, but additionally the Act included a clause which obliged hospitals to provide women with religious and moral instruction. This last measure was quite significant, given how this sanitary legislation

---

68 Paul Mc Hugh, *Prostitution and Victorian Social Reform* (London: Croom Helm, 1980), 41.

was seen as aiming to restore prostitutes and society back to their moral and physical health. Similarly, penalties for prostitutes were doubled and even those who lived within five miles from the subjected districts were liable to arrest if they had been found working in the superintended area during the previous fortnight, bringing the system closer to its European counterparts and to venereal legislation in the colonies. There was a minor amendment in 1868 and, as with the 1864 Act, women were given a certificate when they were cured and released from hospital.[69]

At the time of the second Contagious Diseases Act the London Lock Hospital had already cleaned up its accounts and was going through a period of financial stability. In 1865, new plans had been resolved to build a new wing at Westbourne Green, and on 26th April 1866, the War Office applied for 15 extra beds in the Female Hospital until the building was finished. Later in July the number of Government beds was increased to 80, and a subscription of 3,600 pounds for usual contributors was made to the New Wing, which was opened on 1st June 1867 by the Duke of Cambridge, and named the Prince of Wales Wing. Five beds in the Asylum were also to be taken by the War Office, and the hospital rules were altered to make provision for extra medical staff. In the same fashion and due to the considerable number of new patients and the lack of room in the Chapel, arrangements were made to hold additional services in the wards during the week to provide patients with the religious and moral instruction that the Act demanded. It was also approved that missionaries could visit the Hospital on Sundays as well as the residence of the Chaplain in the grounds. In 1868 the total number of beds required by the Government in the Lock Hospital was 120, and in April 1869 it was arranged that a new ward was to be built, elevating the number to 152.[70]

The logic behind extending the Act to the to the civil population had to be based on a series of reasons such as the presence of similar conditions for

---

69   Howell, *Geographies of Regulation: Policing Prostitution in Nineteenth-Century Britain and the Empire*, 41–42; Sigsworth and Wyke, "A Study of Victorian Prostitution and Venereal Disease", 95.
70   *Patient Records, Correspondence and Plates*, "An Account of the Lock Hospital, from Notes Taken from the Minute Books", MS0022/6/3.

the spread of venereal disease, the universality of the benefits of regulation, the eradication of the problems associated with the "Great Social Evil" and the positive implications both for prostitutes and respectable society. The women under regulation could move out of the trade and have a decent employment, and brothels and all signs of public vice could be eliminated from the streets.[71] This rationale was beneath the creation of the Association for Promoting the Extension of the Contagious Diseases Acts to the Civilian Population (known as the Extensionist Association) in 1866 and the Report produced by the Harveian Medical Society of London in 1867. The Report was made at the request of the International Medical Congress which asked participants for a survey about the incidence of venereal disease and the existing lock facilities in their respective countries. The Committee set up by the Harveian Society discovered that there was not enough lock accommodation and that the incidence of venereal disease in the civilian and military population of Great Britain was alarmingly high, calling for the extension of the system of regulation.[72] As regards the Association, fuelled by the Harveian Report, it was a campaigning pressure group which had an established constituency made of outstanding patrons from the professional and political classes. Amongst its members were prestigious surgeons, doctors, deans and vice-chancellors, and members of the aristocracy. Although there were branches in other cities of England and in Ireland, it was mainly a London-based and Southern English movement, which reflects the geography of the Acts and the location of authority and power. The most contentious group inside the Association was composed of medical men who were venereologists, and among them was William Acton; they aspired to developing sanitary science and state medicine, but they constituted only one third of its members. Aristocratic supporters probably had a greater tolerance of prostitution and disease, and members of the teaching profession would feel the need to protect the morals and health of their young men. The case of the Anglican Church was even

---

71 Howell, *Geographies of Regulation: Policing Prostitution in Nineteenth-Century Britain and the Empire*, 54–55.
72 Walkowitz, *Prostitution and Victorian Society: Women, Class and the State*, 79.

more prominent, and divines were fervent defenders of regulation until at least 1881, as also were many Catholic priests. Similarly, all public authorities like policemen, magistrates or civil servants were in favour of extension. However, they did realise that the movement towards universal regulation had to be gradual, because opposition would be generated. Likewise, the extension of the Acts to the capital would be a far more complicated step which would need exceptional legislation.[73]

The Association's arguments for promoting extension were concerned with the health and well-being of the community due to the infectious nature of venereal disease, which they described as "preying, like a cankerworm, upon our national life, and carrying misery, deformity, and premature death far and wide, throughout all ranks of society, though most palpably and grievously in its lowest ranks".[74] The solution lay in everyone's hands by applying human means to combat the illness and by using the authority of the Government. Their argumentation had again the same logic as that of the London Lock accounts and reports and they resorted to the comparison between venereal disease and other epidemics, fevers and even plagues which had affected cattle to talk about a crusade against vice and immorality and about preventive action. They also claimed the innocence of some of the victims like children and the wives of sinners, and the Christian virtue of charity in favour of the culprits. Other benefits of extension would be the removal of prostitutes from the streets and checking the spread of illness by detaining them, which in some cases might lead to cure and reform.[75] Again, all this reflects the ideology of the 1860s and 1870s behind the control of prostitution and venereal disease.

Thanks to the Extensionist Association's activity, one of its members, Viscount Lifford, called for a Select Committee in the House of Lords to discuss the issue of extending the Acts. After examining 18 witnesses, 17 were in favour of the measure, and the Report was published on 2nd July 1868.

---

73 Howell, *Geographies of Regulation: Policing Prostitution in Nineteenth-Century Britain and the Empire*, 54–61.
74 "Extension of the Contagious Diseases Act of 1866 to the Civil Population". *The Lancet*, July 4, 1868: 21.
75 Ibid., 21–22.

Although the Committee stated that to apply extension was outside its powers, the members agreed that the previous Acts of 1864 and 1866 had been successful from a moral and sanitary point of view. However, they recommended several improvements to the previous legislation: to increase the five-mile limit for subjected districts to avoid prostitutes moving out of it; to allow visiting surgeons to have powers to ask the police to arrest women who did not appear on the appointed day; and to extend the detention of women to nine months if necessary. Additionally, the Committee pointed out that the treatment of children and pregnant women was not adequate, and proposed that children be sent to Industrial Schools to be cured at the expense of their parents, and that pregnant women be permitted to have their confinement at Lock Hospitals in order not to stop their treatment as had been the case so far. Finally, they even suggested a return to the medical examination of men in the armed forces.[76]

Another Select Committee on the 1866 Act in the House of Commons followed, and was set up on 8th June 1869. The Committee consisted of 21 members, and 13 witnesses were interviewed, most of whom had experience in the application of the Act or in issues of public health. They were conscious of the improbability of extending the Acts to the whole country and produced a more cautious report suggesting the Commons improving previous legislation and elaborating a short list of additional districts while establishing another Select Committee to consider further extension. The staff at the London Lock participated in the various Commissions that were established to discuss the extension and application of the Contagious Diseases Acts. As a result, in August 1869, the third Contagious Diseases Act was passed as an amendment to the 1866 one, extending to ten miles the limits of the subjected districts, lengthening the maximum time of detention in hospital to nine months, and allowing the detention of women for up to five days if they were not fit for examination. Visiting surgeons could stop the examination of women after consulting the police, and women were no longer given their certificates of discharge: these were to be kept

---

76 Spongberg, *Feminising Venereal Disease: The Body of the Prostitute in Nineteenth Century Medical Discourse*, 63–64.

by the hospitals to avoid misuse. The application of the Acts was extended to Canterbury, Dover, Gravesand, Maidstone and Southampton, which became subjected districts, remaining so till the laws were suspended in 1883 and repealed in 1886.[77]

During the period that the Contagious Diseases Acts were in operation, the London Lock Hospital received a significantly larger number of female patients coming from the garrison towns where the facilities for women with venereal disease were not ready or where the number of patients exceeded the number of beds available. The peak year was 1868, when 1,133 women were accepted with an average occupation of almost 100 beds a day. Private patients were no longer accepted during this period.[78] In 1866, the London Lock Hospital received patients from the subjected districts of Sheerness, Chatham, Woolwich, Aldershot, Windsor, Greenwich and Canterbury.[79] According to Dr. James Lane, Surgeon to St. Mary's and the Lock Hospital, in 1867 the Government cases came from Woolwich, Chatham, and Aldershot after compulsory inspection. However, the total number of beds available at the time was 130, of which 30 were assigned to women who applied voluntarily to the Hospital in the usual way. The average stay of ordinary cases was 50 days, and that of Government cases was less than 31 days. Cases could be divided into two types: those with syphilis and those with gonorrhoea; syphilis accounted for 80% of the ordinary cases, while in Government cases it did not represent more than 41.5%. According to these data, it seems clear that the incidence and severity of venereal disease on women subjected to regular inspection was less prominent than in women that constituted the regular voluntary cases, who were usually older. The explanation probably lies in the fact that subjected women could not leave the Hospital until a surgeon certified that they were completely clear of the disease, under the threat of imprisonment,

---

77 Mc Hugh, *Prostitution and Victorian Social Reform*, 51–52; Sigsworth, and Wyke, "A Study of Victorian Prostitution and Venereal Disease", 95.
78 Innes Williams, *The London Lock: A Charitable Hospital for Venereal Disease, 1746–1952*, 93–95.
79 Howell, *Geographies of Regulation: Policing Prostitution in Nineteenth-Century Britain and the Empire*, 45.

whereas the ordinary patients not only came to the Hospital when the illness had got to a really serious state but also left the premises at their own request when the most virulent symptoms had disappeared. Nonetheless, when patients under the Acts returned to their old ways, venereal disease appeared again, and sometimes they were readmitted several times to the Hospital, which had not been the common practice before this legislation was passed.[80] Dr. James Lane also mentioned that a large number of patients from the military districts suffered from uterine and vaginal discharges, and that 58% of these women in 1867 and 65% in 1868 had these complaints. They were young girls between 17 and 25 in quite good condition and their affection was totally local with little pain, which he attributed to "the continual irritation and excitement of their generative organs consequent upon their mode of life".[81] The treatment and diagnosis of these women included the use of the speculum and, when there was no "constitutional" fault, the cure could be effected by local application using vaginal injections that the patients themselves could employ; however, if discharges proceeded from the interior of the cervix uteri, the surgeon had to apply through the speculum suitable remedies to the os and cervix. This treatment must have been effective, as women remained healthy for a considerable period of time.[82] Also, rest and regular diet and habits would work to restore them to a healthy condition. Despite all this, Dr. Lane insisted that, without compulsory inspection, many women suffering from gonorrhoea and uterine and vaginal discharges would spread the disease even more alarmingly through contagion, and that prevention was important for detecting the complaint at an early stage. He was clearly in favour of regulation, and insisted that the measure was good for these women who could avoid permanent mutilation and loss of health. He called for greater attention to be paid to the shortage of venereal facilities

---

80 James R. Lane, F.R.C.S., "Remarks on the Cases Admitted into the London Female Lock Hospital during the Year 1867", *The British Medical Journal* 1 (372), February 15, 1868: 139–140.
81 James R. Lane, F.R.C.S., "Notes on the Practice of the London Female Lock Hospital", *The British Medical Journal* 2 (414), December 5, 1868: 592.
82 Ibid., 592.

in London where the number of prostitutes of the worst type, that is, those who consorted with thieves and the like was 6,000 according to police records, and constituted only half the number of the total of women who made their living on the streets. From interviews he had conducted with many women, Lane even claimed that they showed no aversion towards compulsory examination or detention, and were content with the system.[83]

This is the reading that F.B. Smith makes of the application of the Contagious Diseases Acts, which gives some agency to the subjected women who submitted voluntarily to inspection and saw the benefits of treatment for their health and working lives and in contrast with the arguments of the advocates of repeal. Although he talks about the possibility of corruption among magistrates and the police in the application of this legislation, he mentions that the fact that "the Queen's Women" were given clean certificates made them professionals and allowed them to improve their lives. In the same way, under the system many young girls under 16 were returned to their family or friends, or sent to reformatories and asylums, and many women had their names removed from the register when they married or commenced decent employment, having then the opportunity of starting a new life. In contrast with this position, we have the attitude of feminist historians who see the Contagious Diseases Acts as a form of punishment in the brutal and painful treatment that women suffered. In their view, the system did not benefit the prostitutes, who were stigmatised as symbols of immorality and pollution and whose bodies were the focus of control and surveillance, ignoring the role played by men in the spread of disease.[84] Their identities and agency were certainly in many cases erased and subjugated to the medical and moral discourses of the time which produced the power and knowledge that transformed their bodies into "texts of culture" – following Bordo's and Foucault's notions – at the service of the hegemonic ideology of the middle class.

---

83   Lane, F.R.C.S., "Remarks on the Cases Admitted into the London Female Lock Hospital during the Year 1867", 139–140.
84   Spongberg, *Feminising Venereal Disease: The Body of the Prostitute in Nineteenth Century Medical Discourse*, 70–71.

Either way, the consequences of the Acts for the London Lock were of significance with the great increase in the number of patients and the subsequent enlarging of the buildings and fund from Government. As a result, charitable support diminished considerably and the public perception of the Hospital changed: it came to be viewed as a place of punishment and incarceration more than as a place of refuge and cure for the destitute poor with venereal disease. With the Repeal Campaign that ensued, things would change even further, influencing gravely the finances of the Institution.[85]

There were also many elite doctors who were averse to the Contagious Diseases Acts. An important stimulus to fight against regulation came from the 11th Report of the Medical Officer to the Privy Council published by Sir John Simon, already mentioned above, in the *Westminster Review* in 1868. He was very critical of the conclusions of the investigations carried out by the Skey Committee and manifested his opposition to extending the legislation to the rest of the population. This underlined the divergence between government and medical authorities.[86] His arguments were that ratepayers would not be ready to run with the costs of safeguarding the health of their promiscuous neighbours; education for boys of the upper classes should stress moral responsibility in them. From a sanitary point of view, he was ahead of his time in stating that syphilis had lost severity in the 1860s, and that sometimes the illness was not distinguished from other forms of venereal complaints, which led to an overestimate of its incidence.[87]

The Repeal Campaign was born during the Social Science Congress at Nottingham in October 1869, where the creation of the National Anti-Contagious Diseases Acts Association, later known as the National Association for the Repeal of the Contagious Diseases Acts (NA), took shape. The Association established its local branches in 1870. At the beginning, the Association did not accept women, although it quickly changed its policy. Also, a Ladies' National Association (LNA) was founded and

---

85 Innes Williams, *The London Lock: A Charitable Hospital for Venereal Disease, 1746–1952*, 86.
86 Spongberg, *Feminising Venereal Disease: The Body of the Prostitute in Nineteenth Century Medical Discourse*, 75–76.
87 Mort, *Dangerous Sexualities: Medico-Moral Politics in England since 1830*, 70.

based in London – though it had numerous branches throughout the country – under the leadership of some prominent women like Josephine Butler, Harriett Martineau, Elizabeth Wolstenholme, Margaret Tanner, Mary Priestman or Florence Nightingale, and men like James Stansfeld, William Shaen, F.C. Banks, Sheldom Amos or Henry Wilson, overshadowing the repeal activity of the National Anti-Contagious Diseases Acts Association. The LNA was especially strong in the North and the East in the 1870s but the support of membership in the West and South was not as high. There was particularly strong repeal support in Yorkshire and Ireland as well, and Liverpool, Butler's hometown, was a key place in the battle for repeal.[88]

Josephine Butler (1828–1906) became the most visible leader of this crusade. She was born in Dilston, Northumberland, in a middle-class family. Her father was an agricultural reformer and antislavery advocate, and he educated his children in the idea of promoting the spiritual equality of all human beings, implicating them in the political and social questions of their time. She had a close relationship with her mother and sisters and married George Butler in 1851, who gave her his support in all her activities.[89] After tragedy struck their lives with the accidental death of their daughter when they were living in Oxford in 1863, they moved to Liverpool and Josephine began a life of rescue work and philanthropy which put her in contact with prostitution. After visiting the workhouse, she made of her own home a place of refuge for many fallen women. The number of women seeking help was increasingly alarming and Josephine decided to found her Home of Rest, recruiting the help of her recently widowed sister Fanny to look after these "fallen angels".[90] According to her own granddaughter, "her intention was no less than to set right what she considered the unjust relation of women to men as regards moral affairs. It was their equality in everything that she wanted. It was rather the removal of an iniquitous unfairness to

---

88 Howell, *Geographies of Regulation: Policing Prostitution in Nineteenth-Century Britain and the Empire*, 62–63.
89 Walkowitz, *Prostitution and Victorian Society: Women, Class and the State*, 115.
90 Nancy Boyd, *Josephine Butler, Octavia Hill, Florence Nightingale: Three Victorian Women who Changed the World* (London: the Macmillan Press, 1982), 38.

women".[91] She had not been very interested in The Contagious Diseases Acts until her feminist friend, Elizabeth Wolstenholme, invited her to lead the campaign against them in 1869. She took her time to make a decision as her activism would affect her family because the life of a political campaign was hard and dangerous for a middle-class woman. Nonetheless, she counted on the support of her husband, although she would feel the contempt of her peers. Her role in the process of suspension and repeal of the Acts has always been acknowledged by most social historians.[92] There are, however, some academics who consider that her positive role in the campaign has been overestimated and that, occasionally, she behaved in an awkward way. One of these historians defines her as "self-obsessed, histrionic and wilfully uncompromising", and she was not certainly very wise in some of her words and actions.[93]

The majority of women who were on the steering board were of mature age, had the support of their families and were married, and thus they could move around the country and make public speeches on such delicate issues as prostitution, internal examination and venereal disease. Also, as middle-class mothers, they could protect and instruct their fallen working-class sisters. These women shared religious affiliations as well, and they had moved towards feminism through moral crusades like abolitionism and temperance.[94] The Repeal Movement found opposition not only in medical and military environments, but also in Parliament on grounds of immorality. For this reason, repealers used the language of radical dissenting religion, which was a linking nexus between the different groups, as "it offered a set of concepts, a rhetoric of resistance and a strength of moral certainty powerful enough to take on the weight of the medical and political establishment".[95] Butler believed that God had made both man and woman equal on spiritual grounds, but also endorsed

---

91 A.S.G. Butler, *Portrait of Josephine Butler* (London: Faber and Faber, 1954), 56.
92 Nancy Boyd, *Josephine Butler, Octavia Hill, Florence Nightingale: Three Victorian Women who Changed the World*, 39–40.
93 Smith, "The Contagious Diseases Acts Reconsidered", 211.
94 Walkowitz, *Prostitution and Victorian Society: Women, Class and the State*, 118–124.
95 Mort, *Dangerous Sexualities: Medico-Moral Politics in England since 1830*, 69.

some feminist arguments, supporting the idea that there was a connection between unemployment among working-class women and prostitution in her 1869 collection of essays *Woman's Work and Woman's Culture*. She was also in favour of women's education, and in her first pamphlet published in 1868, *The Education and Employment of Women*, she put forward the idea that higher education would provide women with better job opportunities. In fact, women's education was one of her main concerns in the 1860s.[96]

Both Nightingale and Butler saw prostitutes as the victims of Victorian society and the application of the Contagious Diseases Acts; they got involved in the Repeal Campaign between 1870 and 1886, manifesting their opposition to the compulsory inspection of suspected prostitutes and the role of middle-class men in the process. They argued that this practice was discriminatory as men did not have to undergo medical examination. For them, this activity known as "the rape of the speculum" was humiliating for working-class women and sanctioned the existence of prostitution as a vent for male sexual impulses, as Florence Nightingale stated in a letter to her sister, Parthenope Verney, in 1863.[97] In Josephine Butler's own words, "the elevation of impure and unlawful intercourse to the dignity of a recognised traffic under legal regulations, exercises a most baneful influence on the community".[98] And these are some of the arguments that can be found in one of the key elements in the history of the Repeal Campaign: The Ladies' Manifesto, also called the *Women's Protest*, of January 1870. After visiting the subjected districts, Butler drew up this document which included the various arguments against the application of the Contagious Diseases Acts as discriminatory measures against women. The document was signed by very prominent women who were outstanding feminists in many cases, and appeared in the *Daily News* and many other relevant newspapers.[99] The Manifesto consisted of eight points which supported

---

96   Walkowitz, *Prostitution and Victorian Society: Women, Class and the State*, 117.
97   Lynn McDonald, ed., *Florence Nightingale on Women, Medicine, Midwifery and Prostitution* (Ontario: Wilfrid Laurier University Press, 2005), 446.
98   E. Moberly Bell, *Josephine Butler: Flame of Fire* (London: Constable and Co. Ltd., 1962), 90.
99   Ibid., 76–78.

the petition for the abolition of the Acts; according to it, the Acts had been passed in silence, the reputation and security of women was in the hands of the police, the offence was not distinctly established and only women and not men were punished for public vice. They considered that the Acts were "violating the feelings of those whose sense of shame is not wholly lost, and further brutalising even the most abandoned".[100] The success of the Acts was questioned, but the writers were in favour of legislation that worked against immorality and in favour of social reform.

Repealers fought medics on two different fronts: on the one hand, they refuted their statistics that endorsed the improvement of moral and physical health. Here, they published an enormous amount of pamphlets and tracts. On the other, they attacked the ideas of hygiene and sanitation implied in the legislation. Here, they joined moral and feminist discourses together to accomplish an overwhelming critique of male desire; they also attacked the double standard of the Acts and based their strategies on the reform of men's sexuality. Feminists fought to erode the association between active female sexuality and vice, animality and filth, and established the male as the source of contagion and corruption and not the prostitute's body. In this way, middle-class women became agents controlling immorality, safeguarding the purity of the nation through marriage, family and rescue work. They saw prostitutes as victims of "terrible aristocratic doctors" and "debauched aristocrats" and found in reclamation the opportunity for prostitutes to return to their former state of asexual purity. For this reason they developed a punitive attitude to those hardened women who were rebellious and unrepentant.[101] Therefore, the role of purity feminists was associated with women's traditional role to subvert patriarchal power, as it was they, and not their male counterparts who would exert power and control over their working-class sisters. They were their hierarchical superiors, but at the same time they were caring and protective towards young prostitutes. These ideas were also behind many of the activities carried out

---

100 J.E. Butler, *Personal Reminiscences of a Great Crusade* (London: Horace Marshall and Son, 1910), 9–10.
101 Mort, *Dangerous Sexualities: Medico-Moral Politics in England since 1830*, 72–76.

by the London Lock Hospital and Asylum in relation to working-class women who suffered from venereal disease. Feminist leaders also resorted to sensational stories of false entrapment or violation of wombs, presenting women as the inexperienced victims of male desire and medical and police oppression.[102]

The Repeal Campaign also had the support of working-class men and women who wanted to fight to protect their daughters and sisters who were the victims of the Acts and of male lust. Feminists reminded fathers of their protective roles towards their daughters and their patriarchal responsibilities towards their families. Repealers hated the attitude of aristocrats who were in favour of regulation, at least as much as middle-class men.[103] For them, Josephine Butler had really harsh words:

> Those gentlemen who make such a noise about the necessity of prostitution too often forget, I think [sic] that in order to satisfy the necessity the *dishonour of the daughter of the people* is indispensable, for till now none of the worshippers of these medical theories have been found ready to declare willingness that their own daughters should be sacrificed.[104]

Not only working-class men and women but the prostitutes themselves came into the public arena to attend meetings of the LNA throughout the country and to favour a change in the law that would consider them worth protecting and saving. After the publication of the *Protest*, a "Conspiracy of Silence" followed; during four years nothing regarding abolition was published in the national press. As a consequence, the National Association established its own newspaper, *The Shield*, which kept the abolitionists in touch and where Josephine Butler could include her speeches and pamphlets.[105] Another relevant episode was that of the Colchester election of 1870 where Butler organised public agitation against Sir Henry Storks

---

102 Walkowitz, "Male Vice and Female Virtue: Feminism and the Politics of Prostitution in Nineteenth-Century Britain", *History Workshop Journal* 13 (1982): 80–81.
103 Butler, *Portrait of Josephine Butler*, 71–72.
104 Boyd, *Josephine Butler, Octavia Hill, Florence Nightingale: Three Victorian Women who Changed the World*, 78.
105 Moberly Bell, *Josephine Butler: Flame of Fire*, 79–80.

as prospective Liberal MP. The reason was that he was in favour of the Contagious Diseases Acts and came from a colonial regulationist background. Repealers in Colchester had their own candidate, J. Baxter Langley, but the Tory candidate won the election, making evident the abolitionists' capacity to mobilise local opposition.[106]

With the social agitation of the repeal movement and the confrontation between regulationists and repealers, many petitions were sent to Parliament, which finally appointed a Royal Commission at the end of 1870. In 1871 it started to take evidence from a number of prominent witnesses, and Josephine Butler was one of them. The main objectives of the Commission were to find out about the functioning of the Acts, and to determine if the incidence of venereal disease had ameliorated in the subjected districts, and if the treatment of women under the system had been humane. The evidence given by doctors who worked in Lock Hospitals continued to define the prostitute as a pathological creature who was different from the virtuous woman. She still had to be treated as a site of disease and pollution, and syphilis continued to be associated with poverty and immorality.[107] Medics believed that the virulence of venereal disease had diminished since the application of the Acts, and they still recommended the periodical examination of prostitutes and their compulsory treatment. When Josephine Butler gave evidence in front of the Commission, her delivery was a bit disappointing as she proposed very few measures that targeted prostitution and not disease; she suggested punishment for seduction and the reform of the laws of bastardy. Butler supported the idea of voluntary lock hospitals, trusting that women would stay until cured, and proposed to raise the age of consent.[108] Her attitude was defiant, and when she was asked about the cases of abuse against girls committed by the police and if there was any sense of shame left in them, she answered that these fallen

---

106 Howell, *Geographies of Regulation: Policing Prostitution in Nineteenth-Century Britain and the Empire*, 64–65.
107 Spongberg, *Feminising Venereal Disease: The Body of the Prostitute in Nineteenth Century Medical Discourse*, 76–77, 82.
108 Innes Williams, *The London Lock: A Charitable Hospital for Venereal Disease, 1746–1952*, 93.

women could be redeemed and that they had a greater sense of morality than many gentlemen who had recourse to prostitution. She really believed that the power of God lay behind the fight for repeal.[109]

The Report published in the summer of 1871 recommended the suspension of compulsory examination and contained seven minority reports which made conclusions quite confusing and that still supported the double standard like "There is no comparison to be made between prostitutes and the men who consort with them. With the one sex the offence is committed as a matter of gain, with the other it is an irregular indulgence of a natural impulse".[110] The government was reluctant to follow the recommendations of the Royal Commission and there were several attempts to pass a Repeal Bill which were unsuccessful. In 1872, The Home Secretary, H.A. Bruce, introduced a Bill which intended to supersede the Acts, raising the age of consent from twelve to fourteen. However, women soliciting in the streets would be arrested and if found diseased detained in the prison infirmary for up to nine months and brothel-keepers subjected to summary convictions, which meant that regulation was actually extended to the whole country. As a consequence, Josephine Butler manifested her opposition and convinced members of the LNA that the Bill was not good for their cause. Prime Minister Gladstone withdrew it eventually, and new impulse was given to their crusade.[111]

After the failure of the Royal Commission of 1871, repealers began to see the necessity for medical and scientific arguments. At the end of 1874, the National Medical Association for the Repeal of the Contagious Diseases Acts (NMA) was established under the leadership of Dr. John Nevins. Their role in the campaign was fundamental and has been very much neglected by historians. They had their own journal, the *Medical Enquirer*, and became the counterpoint to the regulationist medical press. They advocated personal rights as essential to the social progress of the

---

109   Moberly Bell, *Josephine Butler: Flame of Fire*, 90–91.
110   Ibid., 89.
111   Boyd, *Josephine Butler, Octavia Hill, Florence Nightingale: Three Victorian Women who Changed the World*, 44.

nation and thought that the Acts weakened individual freedom. Another Select Committee was created by the Conservative Government in 1879 to examine the operation of the Acts and decide on their continuance or suspension. James Stansfeld and Harcourt Johnstone, two prominent members of the repeal movement, were appointed, and Nevins claimed that the statistics that presented the decrease of syphilis in the army were not correct, and could not be attributed to regulation but to a natural decline and to better diagnosis and treatment on the part of doctors. Both the *British Medical Journal* and *The Lancet* endorsed the views of pro-regulation doctors, demanding the maintenance of the Acts. After the general election and change of government, hearings were resumed in 1881, and pro-repeal witnesses like Dr. Routh, Dr. Drysdale and Professor Lee continued with Dr. Nevins' case against the Acts.[112]

Josephine Butler gave evidence again to the new Commission in May 1882. However, this time she was more coherent in her arguments about morality and justice, and less aggressive. The Majority Report was signed by nine members of the Commission and the Minority Report by six. In the Majority Report, the old positions of the former Royal Commission were kept, recommending the application of the Acts. By contrast, the Minority Report presented the case against the Acts in a clear and comprehensive way. The National Association fuelled the campaign throughout the country to press Parliament to hear public opinion in favour of abolition, and in April 1883 Stansfeld introduced the motion "That this House disapproves of the compulsory examination of women under the Contagious Diseases Acts", which was approved by Parliament.[113] The longed-for victory had come: the Contagious Diseases Acts were suspended in 1883 but they could not be repealed until 1886. Nonetheless, the system of regulation and compulsory examination and detention continued in the colonies till the end of the century, and many members of the medical profession and the armed forces continued with their demand for re-enactment.

112 Spongberg, *Feminising Venereal Disease: The Body of the Prostitute in Nineteenth Century Medical Discourse*, 85, 90–94.
113 Moberly Bell, *Josephine Butler: Flame of Fire*, 157–163.

The Acts had had several relevant outcomes such as the professionalisation of prostitutes, their mobility in and out of the registered districts, the change in their age spectrum as most of them were now older than in other areas not subjected to regulation, and their segregation to certain neighbourhoods. Some of these shifts had also been observed in other areas which were not under regulation, particularly when talking about the reduction in the number of prostitutes and brothels. Despite repeal and suspension, the ideology behind the Contagious Diseases Acts in terms of moral and physical pollution was to remain throughout the last decades of the nineteenth century, bringing more coercive measures under the new purity politics that emerged, especially after the passing of the Criminal Law Amendment Act in 1885.[114] After their elimination, the London Lock suffered a period of readjustment with a decline in the number of admissions and a drop in Government funding. Subscriptions and donations had fallen but special appeals continued and the money came apparently from the City Livery Companies and the London parishes which continued sending patients and paying for their treatment. Hospital Sunday Collections and Lock Charities and Religious Societies were started, and many changes were brought to the Institution under the impact of the changes seen during the 1880s and 1890s.

---

114   Howell, *Geographies of Regulation: Policing Prostitution in Nineteenth-Century Britain and the Empire*, 66–69.

CHAPTER 5

From Deviancy to Purity: The London Lock Asylum and Moral Reform

As has been stated in Chapter 1, the London Lock Asylum became a prominent feature of the London Lock after its creation in 1787 on the initiative of Rev. Thomas Scott, Chaplain to the Lock Chapel. He proposed the opening of an Institution for girls who, after release from hospital, could not avoid former friends and had given "sufficient proof of sincere repentance". The main aim was to protect them till they could be restored to friends or family, and the community at large "in a way of Industry according to their ability", and to support them even after discharge if they maintained an irreproachable behavior in their new situations in life.[1] At this early stage the Asylum would accommodate up to 20 inmates under the supervision of a Matron and with the support of a separate list of subscribers from that of Hospital, who were mostly ladies, together with Hospital Governors and all the medical staff. A Committee of Governors was in charge of the supervision of the Asylum, but later a Ladies' Committee was established to oversee its management and other practical matters. The staff was reduced to a minimum since penitents did most of the work, as we shall see.[2]

The London Lock became more involved in the reform work that characterised its evolution throughout the nineteenth century at the end of the eighteenth, when reforming disciplinary institutions were born out of the campaigns developed by groups such as the Society for the Promotion of Christian Knowledge (SPCK) and the Society for the Reformation of

---

1   *A Short History of the London Lock Hospital and Rescue Home, 1746–1906* (The Library, Royal College of Surgeons of England, London), 16–17.
2   David Innes Williams, *The London Lock: A Charitable Hospital for Venereal Disease, 1746–1952* (London and New York: Royal Society of Medicine Press Ltd., 1995), 57.

Manners. These institutions promoted confinement and harsh discipline, and worked together for the isolation and identification of deviant members of society. The moral reform of patients had not been the main objective behind the foundation of the London Lock in the first three decades of its existence, but by the 1780s moral improvement became an essential goal with the impulse of the Evangelical Movement at the time of the establishment of the Lock Asylum. However, the gender bias is more than evident in the transformation of the London Lock from a medical institution to one which had the regeneration and the rehabilitation of women as its primary intention.[3] This change in policy has a strong connection with the shift that gender ideology suffered in this period which put the emphasis on domesticity and the separate spheres discussed in Chapter 2. Thus, in the *Account of the Lock Hospital and Asylum of 1834* we can read:

> [...] while the male patients, when cured, return to their former occupations, without any peculiar obstacle to their reformation, most of the women are of that class whose misery and baneful influence have been noticed; many of them have no method of subsistence but by prostitution, and can procure no lodging but in a house of infamy. These have scarcely any alternative, but of starving on the one hand, or returning to their former practices on the other.[4]

In other words, only women were seen as in need of a reform institution. Nonetheless, we must bear in mind that, in line with biblical precept, Evangelicalism believed that women were subordinated to men socially, but, at the same time, serious Christians "firmly believed in the right of all women to salvation" as, following the Scripture, "[...] there is neither male nor female for ye are all one in Christ Jesus" (Gal. 3, 28).[5] So redemption and salvation of fallen women were part of the daily endeavour of the Lock Asylum, but it cannot be claimed that it was the first Charity

---

3   Kevin Siena, *Venereal Disease Hospitals and the Urban Poor: London's Foul Wards 1600–1800* (Rochester: University of Rochester Press, 2004), 182–183.
4   *Account of the Lock Hospital and Asylum, 1834* (The Library, Royal College of Surgeons of England, London), MS0022/3/8.
5   Leonore Davidoff and Catherine Hall, *Family Fortunes: Men and Women of the English Middle Class 1780–1850* (London: Routledge, 1992), 114.

devoted to the indoctrination and reformation of "promiscuous" women, as the Misericordia Hospital and the Magdalene Hospital had already linked moral reform and medical care in the treatment of prostitutes with venereal disease.

The Magdalene Hospital was a model for the Lock Asylum and for all the other homes and penitentiaries that proliferated throughout the nineteenth century, and constituted the first refuge for fallen women. It had been opened in Whitechapel in 1758 by Jonas Hanway. It was later moved to Streatham and admitted female patients between fifteen and twenty who had to be clean of disease. Funding for this charity came from donations from Governors and collections in the Chapel. After that, the first Magdalene Asylums were opened in England, Scotland and Ireland like the Dublin Magdalene Asylum, established in 1767 or the Edinburgh Royal Magdalene Asylum created in 1797. These were succeeded by a series of Penitentiaries and Rescue organisations that founded Magdalene institutions such as the Bristol Female Penitentiary in 1800, Bath Penitentiary in 1805, the London Female Penitentiary Society Refuge in 1807, the London Guardian Society Asylum in 1812, the Liverpool Female Penitentiary in 1810, the Hull Home of Hope in 1811, the Glasgow Magdalene Asylum in 1815, the Devon and Exeter Female Penitentiary in 1819, the Leeds Guardian and the Gloucester Magdalene Asylums in 1821, the York Refuge and the Manchester Asylum for Female Penitents in 1822, the Plymouth Penitentiary in 1832, the London Female Mission in 1836, and the Cambridge Female Refuge in 1838. All of them took their cue from Protestant doctrine and had as their aim the rescue, reclamation and protection of betrayed and fallen women.[6] The Biblical reference to Mary Magdalene is more than obvious and the comparison was established between this sinner prostitute for whom Jesus Christ had shown sympathy and commiseration in the New Testament and these fallen women who were given the chance of redemption and salvation. The idea was to provide them with a family structure that was based on the model of the middle-class home where prostitutes

---

6 Frances Finnegan, *Do Penance or Perish: A Study of Magdalene Asylums in Ireland* (Piltown, Co. Kilkenny: Congrave Press, 2001), 8–9.

would find comfort in an appropriate and domestic environment for their sex, promoting the values of industriousness and religiosity.[7]

In its early stages, the founders of the Magdalene Hospital tried to establish links with the London Lock, so that the moral reformation of its inmates would be accompanied by a physical recovery in a special ward at the Lock Hospital. However, Bromfield set up a Committee which, after careful consideration, did not agree with this idea. Later, after Hanway presented donations from twelve Magdalene Governors, Bromfield asserted that they would receive patients from the Magdalene institution in the usual way. As a consequence, Hanway opened an entirely separate VD hospital, the Misericordia Hospital, to continue with his task of redeeming and saving London's fallen women. Opened in 1774 and located in Goodman's Fields in the East End, a working-class area where the lower type of prostitute was very common, the Misericordia Hospital had a brief existence and appeared in the *Medical Register* till 1783, disappearing probably just a few years later. There are hardly any surviving records, but we know that Hanway hoped to give the new hospital the same characteristics as the Magdalene Hospital, emphasising the principles of work, solitude, prayer and self-reflection, as can be inferred from his *Account of the Misericordia Hospital* published in 1780. The Misericordia was thus the first English institution to unite a venereal hospital with a reform charity, substituting physical punishment with repentance and atonement. The Chaplain was to play a crucial role in the process which was seen as instilling rational capacity and self-restraint in patients through reading divine service, admonishing inmates, preaching in the wards and distributing reading materials and prayer books. Hanway also established a system of letters of recommendation for women who he judged to have benefited from the process of physical and moral rehabilitation sufficiently to become active members of society again. The Misericordia sought to take control over the patients' communications with the outside world as well, supervising correspondence and visitors; it also prevented inmates from having

---

7   Paula Bartley, *Prostitution: Prevention and Reform in England, 1860–1914* (London & New York: Routledge, 2000), 30.

"immoral" conversation or talking about their personal histories. They had to renounce their past when they entered the hospital and make a clear declaration of repentance both to the hospital staff and to their families and friends, forming a new identity. The focus of the Misericordia Hospital's concern was wayward women, so the gender bias was a clear characteristic of the rescue institution.[8]

This idea of transforming women's identities is closely connected with the notion of transgressive interiorities that prevailed in the eighteenth and nineteenth centuries' doctrine of immorality. This doctrine had to do with social practices and technologies of the body associated with power relations. The body becomes a social text where interiorities are recognised and identities can be reformulated and constructed. As stated in Chapter 2, the prostitute's body became a metaphor of dirt, pollution, disorderliness and so on, and "the architecture and design of the body's structures were used to identify and explain innate temperament and the moral faculty".[9] In other words, the causes of immoral behavior were located in certain parts of the body, and in particular in women's bodies as in the case of venereal disease. Thus, prostitutes were identified as carriers of vice, and infectious bodies had to be confined and removed from the community to avoid the spread of contagion among their fellow citizens. This was the ideology behind all Magdalene Asylums. This way of thinking was also class-specific, focusing on the lower orders as naturally predisposed to immorality and promiscuity. This was particularly relevant for the case of lock asylums which established the condition of repentance and remorse for those who had trespassed the boundaries of decency, so that "the expression of embarrassment represented a self-conscious and conscientious being, but more importantly, it demonstrated a 'performative decency', an acknowledgement of normative rules of conduct through the admission of guilt".[10] Prostitutes'

---

8   Siena, *Venereal Disease Hospitals and the Urban Poor: London's Foul Wards 1600–1800*, 206–210.
9   Heidi Rimke, "Constituting Transgressive Interiorities: Nineteenth Century Readings of Morally Mad Bodies", *Violence and the Body: Race, Gender and the State*, ed. Arturo J. Aldama (Bloomington, IN, USA: Indiana University Press, 2003), 250.
10 Ibid., 258.

bodies as texts of culture became the bodies of "the other", according to middle-class ideas of respectability, through their appearance of difference. As a result, the discourses of morality and medicine produced a number of "moral pathologies" which were attributed to those subjects who defied bourgeois values becoming "ungovernable" and showing the existence of pathological interiorities that reflected themselves on the surface of their bodies. In this ideological context, fallen women constituted the target of Magdalene hospitals and asylums.

Consequently, the London Lock Hospital suffered a process of transformation in the 1780s that led to the creation of the Lock Asylum for the Reception of Penitent Women in 1787. The image of prostitutes as victims and with a right to salvation propagated by Evangelicalism and the Clapham Sect was essential for their redemption through a regimen of moral cleansing and discipline. For Evangelicals, ideas of gender division and female subordination were crucial and their belief in the capacity of the individual for change was at the bottom of their rescue work with fallen women. To achieve this aim, prostitutes' working-class identities would be transformed into self-reflective wives and mothers, following the example of the middle class. The Lock Asylum was thus opened to offer women who had been released from the Lock Hospital and showed "sincere repentance" the opportunity to be religiously and morally instructed and to receive vocational training as servants. The logic behind the institution was to train deviant women in an occupation that was appropriate to their station in life and to return them to society as marriageable.[11] To understand the history and work of the Asylum, I will make use of primary sources which have never seen the light in most cases, like Reports and Accounts for the different stages of the institution, the Asylum Regulations and some Asylum Committee minutes that have survived. Of course, all these sources were generated very much by the institution itself; or, even worse, they constituted one precondition for a continued flow of donations, although the Lock Asylum became a more attractive charity for the

---

11   Siena, *Venereal Disease Hospitals and the Urban Poor: London's Foul Wards 1600–1800*, 211–213.

The London Lock Asylum and Moral Reform 131

middle-class than the Hospital itself, and it also had its own sources of income through the needle-work and the laundry-work of the Penitents. However, these sources are far better than nothing, as we can hardly expect many – or, perhaps, any – perspectives to survive from those who had been inmates of the Asylum.

REPORT

OF THE COMMITTEE OF THE

***LOCK HOSPITAL* AND *ASYLUM*,**

READ AT THE PUBLIC MEETING

Held at the Thatched House Tavern, St. James's-street,

ON SATURDAY THE 8th OF JUNE, 1839,

H. R. H. THE DUKE OF CAMBRIDGE
In the Chair.

𝔓imlico:

PRINTED BY J. COWELL, 22, TERRACE, NEAR THE QUEEN'S PALACE.

1839.

Front Cover Report 1839, Cuttings Album, the Library, Royal College of Surgeons of England, MS0022/11.

However, some of the published statistics and objective data about the women can reveal a lot of information about their personal backgrounds, ages, character and origins. Even their lives after they left the Institution can be known, as the Matron and the Committee followed their former inmates' careers, although through the lens of a middle-class bias. As we shall see, some of these women's correspondence with the Matron and the communications of the latter with the middle-class ladies for whom these reformed sinners worked as servants were also set as an example of how successful the Asylum was in its task. Behind this form of propaganda there are details and personal impressions which reflect and reveal some of the feelings of some of these regenerated women. The medical and religious discourses which were underlying these surviving records had a prominent role in moulding working-class prostitutes and fallen women according to middle-class values of respectability and purity, shaping then a gender identity associated with these values. This policy was "unofficial" in the sense that there was no state intervention, as the London Lock was a charitable body dependant on public support, the same as the other Asylums and Penitentiaries. In this respect, it had no powers of enforcement, although other mechanisms such as persuasion or detention were employed. Similarly, the women's reaction was not always coincident with the image propagated by the Lock Reports and Accounts, and the idyllic notions that the Charity pretended to convey were on many occasions contradicted by the women's behaviour and even rebellion in front of these attempts to control their identities and their bodies.

As stated above, the London Lock Asylum was thus heavily modelled on the penitentiary structure of the Magdalene and the Misericordia Hospitals. Like the other Asylums, it was seen as a vital institution for both the physical and moral cure of the nation's sexually deviant, as venereal disease and promiscuity were a plague that had to be controlled. The Lock Asylum focussed on the role of reformation, complementing the work of the Hospital, boosting the charity's finances, and attracting the contributions of new donors who saw their activity with different eyes thanks to the rescue work that was being accomplished.[12] According to Siena, the archives for the Lock Asylum in the eighteenth century are quite incomplete and the decade of the 1790s is almost undocumented, but there are a number of surviving records for the first two years of the Institution. We know that women were prepared for

---

12 Donna Andrew, "Two Medical Charities in Nineteenth-Century London: The Lock Hospital and the Lying-In Charity for Married Women", *Medicine and Charity before the Welfare State*, ed. Jonathan Barry and Colin Jones (London, Routledge: 1991), 94.

work and domesticity via spinning and sewing; inmates received religious instruction and were encouraged to self-reflection through silence and the visits of the Chaplain in the morning and in the evening. They also attended service in the chapel. Penitents had to wear uniforms and were not allowed to have any contact with other inmates or with their families except with the permission and in the presence of the Matron, under whose care were their personal belongings. The Matron had to observe and check the women's behaviour very closely and present a weekly report to the Board which participated actively in their control, perhaps partly because the number of women in the Asylum was very small in its early years.[13]

The Asylum Regulations in the nineteenth century which have survived are those for 1824, 1840 and 1890. Through them, we can obtain an important amount of useful information regarding the functioning of the institution and the character both of inmates and of those who were in charge of its management. However, we must always bear in mind the middle-class bias of these sources, as the voices of the women themselves can never be heard in the surviving archives, except via a handful of exceptional incidents. The three sets of regulations have several aspects in common, with very slight differences, establishing the official mechanisms for admittance and refusal, as well as for release and provision for the future of these women who were called *Female Penitents*. They also established the various rules to be applied to the inmates and the aims and tasks connected with the Charity. In the three documents the beneficiaries of the activities were clearly stated; for example, in the Asylum Regulations for 1840 (revised in 1848) that are part of a manuscript containing the Laws of the London Lock Hospital and Asylum, printed by Chapmans of Star Street, Paddington, the following can be read: "The object of the Institution is to afford a refuge to such of the Female Penitents of the Lock Hospital, as appear sincerely desirous of quitting their evil courses".[14] This sentence plainly establishes

---

13   Siena, *Venereal Disease Hospitals and the Urban Poor: London's Foul Wards 1600–1800*, 216–217.
14   *Laws of the London Lock Hospital and Asylum, Revised (1840), 1848*, The Library (Royal College of Surgeons of England, London), MS0022/5/2.

that the place had been designed as a home of refuge for the fallen who had made the resolution of leaving their former "evil courses" and who had been patients at the Lock Hospital before. Later in the Regulations we can read:

> No females shall be admitted into this Asylum, but those of the Patients of the Lock Hospital, whom the Chaplain, after careful examination, shall report to be proper objects of the Charity – and such will be considered only admissible *immediately* upon their discharge from the Hospital.[15] (Italics in original)

This means that the women had to show sincere repentance and be free from venereal disease to be accepted. It was the Chaplain who was in charge of evaluating the applicant and of deciding if she was an appropriate object for the Charity and had an adequate inclination towards reform. Women could be admitted only once, and the fact that they had to join the Asylum immediately after release from Hospital is significant, as there could be no room for physical or moral corruption. No pregnant women were accepted either; if they applied, they were sent to the workhouse and were only later admitted if they left the baby in the workhouse after confinement.

The way the Institution was governed changed somewhat through the nineteenth century. At the beginning, the management of the Charity was entrusted to a Committee of Governors that was elected annually and had the support of a number of Ladies who superintended the domestic arrangements. Later, in 1847, the Charity was run by the Chaplain and a Ladies' Committee that would meet on the third Thursday of every month in the Vestry of the Chapel. Arrangements would be made so that one lady of the Committee would visit the Asylum at least once a week. By the end of the century the Chaplain and the Committee of Ladies were still in charge of the internal management of the place, but their actions were "subject to confirmation by the Board".[16] The Committee had powers to propose a new member for election by the Board, to form a Subcommittee

---

15 Ibid., MS0022/5/2.
16 *Laws of the London Lock Hospital and Asylum (Rescue Home) 1890* (The Library, Royal College of Surgeons of England, London), MS0022/5/11. This last version of the London Lock regulations was printed by Burt and Sons, 58, Porchester Road, Bayswater, W.

to receive new inmates and confer with the Matron, and to select a suitable candidate when a new Matron was needed. All the minutes and proceedings of Asylum Committee meetings had to be kept in a book provided for that purpose that was submitted to the Board of Governors for their inspection, and this practice was a constant feature throughout the century.

Once an inmate of the Lock Hospital was accepted as a Penitent of the Asylum, she had to go through a probationary period: "The first two months after the admission of a woman into the Asylum, shall be considered a time of probation, and she shall not be fully or finally admitted, until a report of her exemplary conduct, during that period, has been made to the Weekly Committee".[17] Therefore, during this time, the behaviour of the candidate was carefully checked and she was kept in isolation. She had to conduct herself in an appropriate way and if she showed insolence or discontent, her full admission was suspended.[18] When the probationary period was over, the Penitent had to remain in the Asylum for about two years. This was the average length of time that middle-class reformers considered sufficient for the transformation of these women into decent working-class members of society after instruction and indoctrination. This practice was retained throughout the century as was the ideology behind the Charity. Thus, in the *Cuttings Album*, there is an extract from the Annual Report of the Lock Hospital and Asylum of 1860 where it can be read that "The Lock Asylum is intended for the reception of those females, who, after having been discharged cured from the Lock Hospital, desire to give up their evil courses and connections, as to become respectable members of society". And later it is stated that Penitents were "clothed, boarded, and instructed for two years, (many of them being unable to read when admitted) which is found to be a time sufficient to test their sincerity".[19]

17 *Account of the Lock Hospital and Asylum, 1837* (The Library, Royal College of Surgeons of England, London), MS0022/3/8.
18 *Lock Asylum Committee (1836–1842)* (The Library, Royal College of Surgeons of England, London), MS0022/1/4.
19 *Extract from the Annual Report of the Lock Hospital and Asylum, 1st January, 1860, Cuttings Album* (The Library, Royal College of Surgeons of England, London), MS0022/11.

For instance, the declaration that inmates were required to sign to enter the York Refuge – another Asylum for female penitents established in York in 1822 – was extremely significant and expressed the degree to which these girls were required to abandon their previous identities and complied with middle-class values of submission and discipline:

> I am wishful to abandon my sinful life
> And by God's grace lead a better.
> I am willing to remain two years in the Home.
> I will do my best to conform
> To the rules and discipline of the Home.[20]

This declaration is one more manifestation of the way in which these places of seclusion complied with what Foucault defines as the power relations that pervade societies. According to him, bodies acquire significance within the different discourses of an age, and a particular discourse can be defined as a way of describing, defining, classifying and thinking about people, things, and even knowledge and abstract systems of thought. Specifically, in the case of the London Lock Hospital and Asylum, these power/knowledge relations are part of spatial relations that assign a specific place to different bodies in the medical and religious discourses, depending on their gender and class and using binary codes such as fallen/unfallen, decent/corrupted, working-class/middle-class, industrious/idle, submissive/ungovernable, etc. Thus, in his first volume of *The History of Sexuality* (1990), Foucault asserts that power is exercised in what he calls its "capillary forms", that is, through multiple and complex ways, and not by individuals or single groups; rather, he talks of various and shifting positions of power and resistance within a network of relations.[21] In the London Lock, these capillary forms of power are present through a whole network of middle-class reformers, Evangelicals and a system of isolation, confinement and indoctrination of fallen women. Similarly, in his *Discipline and Punish* (1979),

---

20 Frances Finnegan, *Poverty and Prostitution: A Study of Victorian Prostitutes in York* (Cambridge: Cambridge University Press, 1979), 20.
21 Michel Foucault, *The History of Sexuality: Volume I, An Introduction*, trans. Robert Hurley (London: Penguin Books, 1990), 92–98.

Foucault argues that power is primarily exerted on the body and that the model has moved from physical punishment and violence to disciplining bodily actions through knowledge within the different discourses of an age, and through institutions like prisons, hospitals, asylums, etc. Therefore, disciplinary power has become the most efficient and economical way of producing docile and useful bodies, and this was the idea behind the London Lock Asylum.

In this context, the York Refuge functioned in a very similar way to the London Lock Asylum and other institutions of the same kind throughout the country. In both charities, discipline was an essential part of the inmates' routine. The Penitents' behaviour was monitored by the Matron, who had a fundamental role and a very close relationship with the girls, even after they left the Institution, as we shall see. Subordination to rules of conduct started with daily tasks that were quite the same in all the asylums and refuges: the women had to get up very early, start work and then take part in family worship before breakfast; they resumed work till dinner and again after it, and, when supper was finished, there was family worship again. There was always a time of the day devoted to lessons and Bible reading, and the working day lasted no less than ten hours.[22] No direct references can be found in the sources for the Lock Asylum to the Penitents' meals, but there are several examples of diets for the Lock Hospital, so that it can be deduced that they were similar. For instance, in the Glasgow Magdalene Asylum we know that breakfast consisted of porridge; and in the Edinburgh Magdalene Asylum meals were elaborated following the Ladies Committee's advice who recommended cheap dishes and made suggestions like "substituting rice and barley porridge for bread", following the advice of a recipe book published by the Society for Bettering the Condition of the Poor.[23] One of the diets for the Lock Hospital has been described in Chapter 3 and another example of the meals that Patients used to have can be found in the diets included in the Rules for 1814:

---

22 Finnegan, *Poverty and Prostitution: A Study of Victorian Prostitutes in York*, 79–80.
23 Linda Mahood, *The Magdalenes: Prostitution in the Nineteenth Century* (London & New York: Routledge, 1990), 79.

A Table of Diet for the Patients

Low Diet

Breakfast	Water-gruel, Sage or Balm Tea
Dinner	Broth 1 Pint
Supper	Milk Pottage 1 Pint

Milk Diet

Breakfast	Water-gruel or Balm Tea
Dinner	Pudding
Supper	Milk Pottage 1 Pint

Full Diet

Breakfast	Milk Pottage, Water-gruel, Sage or Balm Tea	
Dinner	Sunday	Pudding
	Monday	1 Pound of Meat each
	Wednesday	" " " " "
	Friday	" " " " "
	Tuesday	1 Pint of Broth each
	Thursday	" " " " "
	Saturday	" " " " "
Supper	Milk Pottage, Butter or Cheese	

A Loaf of Bread 14 Ounces, and a Quart of Small Beer[24]

There was a division between "Low Diet", "Milk Diet" and "Full Diet", probably in connection with the surgeons' directions, according to the different medical situations of the patients. There was no fish or chicken except when an indication appeared that these should be included in the diet "at the expense of the Charity". Any of these diets were, by the standards of the time, varied and abundant although one can discern a grievous lack of vegetables and of what, since the 1930s, would be called vitamin C.

---

24   *An Abstract of the Rules and Orders for the Government of the Lock Hospital, near Hyde-Park Corner, Instituted July 4, 1746, for the Relief of Venereal Patients only*, 1814 (The Library, Royal College of Surgeons of England, London), MS0022/5/3.

Similarly, water-gruel, broth, milk pottage, pudding and meat were regular at meals. Bread and beer were also present.[25]

In the Asylum Regulations for 1824 one of the rules referring to the inmates establishes that "The design of their being received is to maintain and protect them until they can be restored either to their friends or to the community at large, in a way of honest industry, according to their ability". That they had to be religiously instructed was added to the 1840 and 1890 Asylum Regulations. The aim behind this training was to produce a "highly-skilled and well-disciplined industrial workforce", together with domestic servants for middle-class households in respectable positions.[26] In the same fashion, with their housework inside the Asylum and the needle-work they did, they could contribute to their maintenance and not be a burden on the Institution. A list of the prices of the needle-work done at the Lock Asylum of around 1844 has survived where their services and rates were described:

Gentlemen's shirts	from 2s. 6d. to 4s. 0d.
Night Shirts	from 1s. 9d. to 2s. 6d.
Gentlemen's collars	from 0s. 4d. to 0s. 8d.
Flannel Waistcoats	from 1s. 0d. to 2s. 2d.
Cravats and silk pocket handkerchiefs	from 0s. 11/2d to 0s. 3d.
Drawers	from 1s. 0d. to 1s. 8d.
Boys' shirts	from 1s. 9d. to 2s. 0d.
Chemises	from 1s. 6d. to 3s. 0d.
Night Do	from 1s. 6d. to 3s. 6d.
Children's chemises	from 0s. 9d. to 1s. 0d.
Pinafores	from 0s. 3d. to 0s. 9d.
Petticoats	from 1s. 0d. to 2s. 6d.

25 Ibid., MS0022/5/3.
26 Mahood, *The Magdalenes: Prostitution in the Nineteenth Century*, 86.

Pockets .... 0s. 6d.

Dressing Gowns .... from 1s. 6d. to 3s. 6d.

Table Cloths... from 0s. 4d. to 0s. 8d.

Table napkins, per dozen.................................. from 1s. 3d. to 1s. 6d.

Towels, per dozen.. from 1s. 3d. to 1s. 6d.

Sheets, per pair .... from 0s. 9d. to 2s. 0d.

Pillow cases, per pair... from 0s. 6d. to 0s. 10d.

Hemming Muslin and Cambric, per yard....... 0s. 1d.

Marking, per letter... 0s. 01/4d.[27]

Another source of income was laundry-work that was perceived as a cleansing ritual and was associated with the moral function that work and discipline had inside the Asylum. On a spiritual level, through this activity "women could do penance for their past sins and purge themselves of their moral contagion".[28] Their clients were middle-class women who saw this transaction as a way of contributing to the reformation and salvation of these girls. As late as 1888, publicity for the Asylum Laundry, known as the Westbourne Green Laundry by that time, asserted that inmates were prepared for that class of washing which would probably imply hard physical work as a way to expiate their sins. It boasted good references and proclaimed that "No chemicals are used in the Laundry, and a large drying-ground is attached".[29] With the use of photographs at the end of the century, the Reports began to include pictures of the Asylum and especially of women doing the laundry-work. The propagandistic effect was probably high, and the aim was to obtain resources for the running of the Charity

---

27 *Cuttings Album* (The Library, Royal College of Surgeons of England, London), MS0022/11.
28 Judith R. Walkowitz, *Prostitution and Victorian Society: Women, Class and the State* (Cambridge: Cambridge University Press, 1991), 221.
29 *London Lock Hospital and Asylum. Report for 1888* (The Library, Royal College of Surgeons of England, London), MS0022/4/2.

that would take women off the streets and keep the public sphere clean. As a result, discipline was imposed to produce useful and docile bodies and to exercise power in a Foucauldian sense. Laundry-work became a symbol of purification for Penitents in Asylums not only in the English system, but also in the Irish and Scottish ones.

The first references to Penitents in the nineteenth century can be found in the Lock Asylum Committee minutes for 1836–1842 that include some entries for patients for 1824, apparently written by the Matron in charge of them – a Mrs. Martha Sterling according to the archives. The rest of the manuscript contains the Asylum Committee minutes of the board that met regularly once a week, dealing mainly with financial matters, although there are some interesting remarks that can give important information about how the Asylum worked. Nonetheless, the women's voices can never be heard directly in the sources. Nine women are mentioned, with ages ranging from 10 to 24, who are depicted as having many aspects in common connected with their behaviour and daily work, mainly focused on needle-work. This is the only time in the sources that we know their names, Ann Hawkins, Mary Sparks, Sarah Spicer, Sarah Gibbon, Sarah Gibbs, Ann Hewitt, Sophia Hall, Ann Carter and Eliza Edwards, but we cannot learn about their thoughts. The most common characteristics attributed to these girls, at least by the Matron, were their idleness, ignorance and inadequate behaviour. For example the girl of ten is described as a poor child that "when first received into the House possessed a perverse temper with many improper habits".[30] It is difficult to ascertain what "improper habits" meant exactly, but they could refer to sexual misconduct and even lesbianism. The majority of them were illiterate and expressions like "ignorant of every kind of useful knowledge", "weak understanding", "slow improvement" or "exceedingly ignorant" were applied to the inmates in the entries for 1824.

As far as instruction and education were concerned, the Penitents were taught their position in the social hierarchy and to accept it and respect their superiors, using the Bible as the primary text and emphasising

---

30 *Lock Asylum Committee (1836–1842)*, MS0022/2/1/4.

"female inferiority, abnegation and duty".[31] Apart from being prepared for professions such as servants, laundresses and needlewomen that were adequate to their station in life, these fallen women received religious instruction through assembling for family prayer and the reading of the Scriptures every morning and evening, receiving the visits of the ministers in their wards and attending the services of the Chapel twice every Sunday. Likewise, the Ladies who frequently visited them undertook the office of teaching them.[32] Thereby, at the Lock Asylum they received lessons in reading and writing, and later in the century, in geography, arithmetic, music and other subjects, which meant a break from routine. However, from the description the Matron gives of the inmates in 1824, they could not have been very clever and must have lacked all basic principles and knowledge. This information can throw some light on the way the low orders of society were perceived as ignorant and morally corrupted by the middle classes; they were seen as indolent and responsible for their own situation. The economic position in which many working-class families found themselves where all the members had to work to survive was not considered a determining factor by many social reformers, and also the fact that many children of the poor did not have access to education was ignored. Another important aspect of Victorian middle-class discourses on sexual deviancy is the connection that was established between lack of morals and imbecility and, as a consequence, many young girls who were mentally retarded were confined in these institutions, as possibly in some of the 1824 entries. This was also the case with Irish Asylums, but these suffered a process of transformation due to the influence of Catholic ideology that will be discussed later in this chapter.

As with the female patients at the Lock Hospital, the inmates of the Lock Asylum were sometimes women that had been prostitutes, or women that had been seduced and had got pregnant, or even women who

---

31 Mahood, *The Magdalenes: Prostitution in the Nineteenth Century*, 83.
32 *Report of the Lock Hospital, Asylum, and Chapel, 1853* (The Library, Royal College of Surgeons of England, London), MS0022/4/2.

had come from the countryside and had been in service in a middle-class household. Many were destitute and "had lived in vicious courses of various kinds" but all of them showed symptoms of "unfeigned repentance".[33] In my view, the identity of these girls was subjugated by a process of "ritual humiliation" that destroyed their femininity. The domestication of these fallen women was also seen in their uniforms which represented their belonging to a community of "reforming penitents" who had abandoned their past existence and had suppressed their sexuality.[34] There is no allusion to the uniform in the London Lock Asylum Regulations but we know that inmates had to wear it, because in the Annual Account for 1888 when it comes to the report on the Charity it is stated that "For the sake of health, cleanliness, and convenience, a special costume is worn by the girls, but they do not object to this, and know that they are at perfect liberty to have their own clothes back, and to leave at any time if they wish".[35] We also know that uniforms were worn in the York Refuge and the Glasgow Magdalene Asylum, as well as in the Irish Magdalene institutions.

In the case of Irish society, we know that an emerging Catholic middle class was leading the process of modernisation and progress that impregnated the nation's identity, spreading notions of moral and social respectability. It seems that Irish Asylums were the response to the high levels of prostitution in Irish society and reflected the involvement of women in philanthropy work. The first Protestant and Catholic Asylums in Ireland were run by lay women with the support of Committees made up of male and female governors and relied on donations and legacies like the London Lock. Later, by the 1830s, female religious congregations began to assume the control of the Catholic ones. Whereas the

---

33 *An Account of the Nature and Intention of the Lock Asylum, for the Reception of Female Penitents when discharged from the Lock Hospital: with an Abstract of the Accounts, from the first Institution, to LADY-DAY, 1833. Also the Code of the Regulations, with a List of Benefactors and Subscribers* (The Library, Royal College of Surgeons of England, London), MS0022/3/8.
34 Bartley, *Prostitution: Prevention and Reform in England, 1860–1914*, 37–39.
35 *London Lock Hospital and Asylum. Report for 1888*, MS0022/4/2.

Protestant institutions closed by the beginning of the twentieth century, most Catholic ones remained open well into the 1990s and represent nowadays one of the most shameful episodes in the history of Irish Catholicism. Thus, the first religious orders that took the control of Irish Magdalene Asylums were the Sisters of Mercy and the Sisters of Charity. Nuns had already been involved in the working of other charity organisations such as orphanages, asylums for the blind, the elderly and the mentally ill. Their power was increased by the Reformatory Act of 1858 and the Industrial Schools Act of 1868, and with a growing atmosphere of morality and respectability in the country. By the middle of the century two French religious orders, the Sisters of Our Lady of Charity of Refuge and the Sisters of Our Lady of the Good Shepherd of Angers got involved in Irish reform work.[36] Irish Magdalene institutions started to work with rules similar to the English ones: silence and prayer were imposed on inmates who had to wear a uniform and short hair and their daily routine consisted in sewing and laundry work. Unlike inmates in the English ones, inmates had to adopt new names and with that the transformation of their identities was complete. But they did not suffer the classification according to their level of depravity that English institutions exerted on girls.[37] In contrast with English asylums, after a period when only prostitutes were admitted, as the nineteenth century progressed, many other types of women were retained on the premises, like single mothers, "promiscuous" women, victims of sexual abuse, women abandoned by their families or employers, and even those who were mentally deranged. With the development of a system of parish clergy, the Catholic Church began to promote a society that put the emphasis on the value of women's modesty and identified the domestic private sphere with the ideal of the nation as a proper family. In this atmosphere where moral and economic interests were prevalent, human sexuality was monitored and supervised, focusing especially on the single mother who carried with

---

36 James M. Smith, *Ireland's Magdalene Laundries and the Nation's Architecture of Containment* (Manchester: Manchester University Press, 2008), 24–25, 28–29.
37 Finnegan, *Do Penance or Perish: A Study of Magdalene Asylums in Ireland*, 22–23.

her illegitimate son the stigma of a social stain, becoming an outcast.[38] Inside Irish asylums, nuns represented authority and the model to follow, whereas in English institutions it was the Matron who had that role. As a consequence, the same hierarchical structure of power was implemented in Irish asylums in a Foucauldian sense, making of them communities of marginalised women. The time of detention in the nineteenth century averaged a few weeks, ranging from a few days to two or three years but, as the century progressed, there were many instances of women penitents who had shown what was seen as outstanding behaviour and became Consecrated Penitents. Most of these were teenagers or in their forties or older and decided to remain in the asylum for life; their main function was to help the Sisters with the other inmates, becoming intermediaries and surveillants. Finally, and in contrast to English institutions, Ireland's Magdalene asylums might admit the same women several times in the hope that they would ascend up a succession of stages, seen as their journey to redemption and spiritual salvation.[39]

In the 1830s the number of women staying in the London Lock Asylum was certainly small, oscillating between 16 in 1835 and 1838, 12 in 1836, 18 in 1837, and 14 in 1839. These figures would vary at the different stages as we shall see, but their final destination was respectable service, their friends, other hospitals, their workhouse parish, and some even died in the house. Another important feature of these years is that quite an important number of them left the Institution for several reasons like eloping, expressing their desire to leave the house or because of being dismissed for bad behaviour. This tendency will remain a constant feature of the Charity throughout the nineteenth century. It remains in tension with the insistence in the Reports and Accounts on the success of reform-work with women who had been the "pests of society".[40]

38 Smith, *Ireland's Magdalene Laundries and the Nation's Architecture of Containment*, 26–27, 30–32.
39 Finnegan, *Do Penance or Perish: A Study of Magdalene Asylums in Ireland*, 130–131, 145.
40 *An Account of the Lock Hospital; to Which is Added an Account of the Lock Asylum, 1837*, MS0022/3/8.

By the middle of the 1840s, the number of women in the Asylum was 43, and most of them were in their late teens or early twenties, so they were very young and malleable. However, two women were twenty-seven and one was ten and almost a child by Victorian standards. Most of them lacked parental references, as they had no parent or only one.[41] Their numbers varied throughout the century, but their features remained as the prevalent characteristics of Asylum inmates, as we shall see. The increase in the number of Penitents from the 1840s onwards can be attributed to the fact that the new building in Westbourne Green was opened in 1842, but the same spirit was kept in the process of saving fallen women's souls. This is exemplified in the inaugural sermon given by the Chaplain, Rev. James Gibson:

> "O Lord Jesus Christ who did'st come to seek and to save that which was lost, and did graciously say to the trembling culprit 'Neither do I condemn thee, go and sin no more', look down, we beseech Thee, with an eye of pity on the inmates of this Asylum. Grant that they who were as sheep going astray, may be brought back to Thee, the Shepherd and Bishop of their souls, that hearing Thy voice and following Thee, Thou mayest give unto them eternal life and that they never perish. Grant this, O Lord, for Thine own name's sake, to whom, with the Father and the Holy Spirit, be all honour and glory, now and forever, Amen".[42]

The parable of the Good Shepherd is part of the argument to keep an institution like this open, together with the idea of sympathy and compassion towards women who had gone astray.

Many of the traits that have featured in descriptions of English and Irish Magdalene Asylums can be applied to the system of penitentiaries that were run throughout the country in the nineteenth century. They were first run by men and were linked to the Established Church, but from the 1840s most of them were under the management of Anglican nuns. The two most important orders that operated what were known as

---

41   *Cuttings Album*, MS0022/11.
42   *Patients Records, Correspondence and Plates, An Account of the Lock Hospital, from notes taken from the Minute Books* (The Library, Royal College of Surgeons of England, London), MS0022/6/3.

"Houses of Mercy" were the community of St. Mary the Virgin and the community of St. John Baptist. Despite their punitive name, Anglican penitentiaries were intended to be reform institutions that worked with fallen women to rehabilitate them on a voluntary basis and to transform them from sexually deviant to socially respectable women. Under the category of fallen women not only prostitutes were included but also any woman who had had sexual intercourse before marriage. This meant that kept mistresses, abused children, victims of incest or rape or simply women who had been thieves or alcoholics were candidates for these places of confinement. Incest was quite common in Victorian homes, according to the records and the casebooks of these Houses of Mercy, as also the rape of servants. Most women were labourers' daughters; many were motherless, had been servants in London and had been in prostitution for less than a year. They were in their late teens or early twenties and showed low levels of literacy. Penitents were expected to remain in the institutions for about two years, but in contrast with the London Lock Asylum no applicant was ever refused admission, although they had an interview with the Mother Superior and the younger the sinner the more malleable she was.[43] The same as happened with many institutions as the century progressed: attempts were made to classify inmates but, sooner or later these places became specialised in the types of inmates they accepted. Inside them, women did laundry and domestic work and were subjected to a strict discipline, the same as the nuns themselves. Penitents were trained for service, teaching and nursing, and received an education which consisted in reading and writing and arithmetic; they might receive good references in order to obtain a position and a complete outfit upon leaving, and could keep in touch with their children if they had any because some sisterhoods also ran orphanages.

Although some inmates absconded, Penitentiaries were open institutions and the only punishment that refractory women received for their behaviour was exclusion. But nuns disciplined inmates through a system of

---

43 Susan Mumm, "'Not Worse than Other Girls': The Convent-based Rehabilitation of Fallen Women in Victorian Britain", *Journal of Social History* 29, 3 (1996): 527–532.

"marks" that they could lose or gain and then promotion through the ranks. Therefore, there were many similarities between Anglican Penitentiaries and Irish Magdalene Asylums, probably because of the religious affiliation of those in charge of the institutions. Both Catholic and Anglican nuns believed in the transformation of women sinners at three levels: bodies, minds and souls.[44] Another common feature between Houses of Mercy and Irish Magdalene Asylums was the idea that the coexistence of middle-class or even upper-class women – the nuns – and working-class prostitutes was a successful approach to reform work, since religious women could be a very positive influence on fallen women, resorting to the gospel to justify this otherwise awkward cohabitation. What was new about Anglican sisterhoods is that they also advocated the raising of male moral standards, overlapping with feminists of the last decades of the nineteenth century who wanted to purify the public space corrupted by men. They took their ideas about reform work to the extreme, allowing women who had been prostitutes to become nuns after their sins had been removed through repentance, accomplishing a radical transformation both on a social and spiritual level. The communities themselves believed that about two thirds of their penitents were successful in their process of reform;[45] again, these figures must be interpreted in a cautious way as the nuns' bias was present in these appreciations.

Returning to the London Lock Asylum, if we focus our attention on the Reports and Accounts for the 1850s we have again the valuable information from Rev. Hind – the Assistant Chaplain at the time – on patients and penitents. The number of patients admitted from the Lock Hospital into the Lock Asylum increased significantly, being some examples of the number of Penitents on the premises the following: 60 Penitents, for instance, in the year 1856, 42 in 1857, or 52 in 1858. The ideology and the workings of the institution had not changed very much during these years: women were occupied as servants, laundresses and

---

44 Mumm, "'Not Worse than Other Girls': The Convent-based Rehabilitation of Fallen Women in Victorian Britain", 535–537.
45 Ibid., 528–529, 540.

needle-women; they had to enter a probationary department where they had to show tokens of their sincerity and repentance. Their moral and religious improvement was the main aim of the charity "to deepen penitential impressions" on its inmates, with their instruction in reading and writing as another priority.[46] Hind alludes on several occasions to the success of the reform work done by the Ladies and the Matrons in charge of keeping the discipline and preparing former sinners to return to society as useful members. In his words, the Establishment was engaged in "seeking to convert sinners from the error of their ways – to the gracious and loving care of Him who came to seek and to save that which was lost".[47]

The years immediately prior to the passing of the three Contagious Diseases Acts and the years of the application of the Acts themselves brought significant changes to the workings of the London Lock Asylum. During this period the Asylum received cases from the Government as well as those who came from the Lock Hospital voluntary wards. The Government paid for the beds in the Asylum for the garrison-town women prostitutes under compulsory inspection.[48] As has been stated in Chapter 4, the number of women admitted into the Lock Hospital as a result of the implementation of the Contagious Diseases Acts increased considerably, thanks to the official cases and the funding from the Admiralty and War Office, and this implied that the number of women in the Asylum augmented. For example, during the years 1868, 1869, 1870 and 1871, the number of patients admitted into the Asylum was 293. There are also some notes of selected cases from the Asylum for these years with the names of the Penitents omitted but with their initials included, probably written by the Matron – a Mrs. Hurd according to the archives. This is again another example of direct references to Penitents in the Asylum which contain both objective and subjective

---

46   *Report of the Lock Hospital, Asylum and Chapel, 1853*, MS0022/4/2.
47   *Report of the Lock Hospital, Asylum and Chapel, 1858* (The Library, Royal College of Surgeons of England, London), MS0022/4/2.
48   Innes Williams, *The London Lock: A Charitable Hospital for Venereal Disease, 1746–1952*, 95.

impressions about them. Their ages oscillated between their late teens and early twenties once more, but there was also a child of 13 and a woman of 25. Many of them were orphans and had led an immoral life for a short time. Most of them came from London and the vicinities of the Lock Hospital from places such as Kensington, Marylebone, Bloomsbury, Greenwich – this was a Government case –, Chelsea, St. John's Wood, Drury Lane, Paddington, and Edgware Road. Some of them had been working in brothels or on the streets, but there was one who had "been upon the stage of the Metropolitan Music Hall".[49] One came from a workhouse and another from Dorchester; another one came under the recommendation of the Marquis of Townshend.[50]

A similar situation can be found at the Glasgow Magdalene Asylum where 109 women had been admitted in 1863, although the system of inspection and control of prostitutes and fallen women in Scotland was different from the English one. Most women in the Glasgow Institution shared many of the features and backgrounds of Penitents in the London Lock Asylum. A large proportion of them were orphans, they lacked proper work or suitable means of subsistence and they had a close relation with vice. They came from the "lower orders of society", but the Magdalene Institution had a long history in the rescue of fallen women. The original Magdalene Asylum had opened in 1812 in response to a growing preoccupation regarding prostitution, venereal disease, and the moral health of the country. In 1863, The Directors of the Institution thought that these women could be redeemed and saved from their immoral life and a more than probable early death. Under the term "prostitute", other types of women were included such as single mothers, socialists, or mill girls who "had fallen". However, after 1859 the Magdalene Asylum transformed into

---

49 The music hall became a popular entertainment for the working classes in the last decades of the nineteenth century, but it was also a place for vile company. It was a business that proliferated through London and other big cities in the United Kingdom. Many prostitutes found their clients during stage performances among members of the audience.

50 *Report of the Lock Hospital and Asylum for the Years 1868, 1869, 1870, 1871* (The Library, Royal College of Surgeons of England, London), MS0022/4/2.

The London Lock Asylum and Moral Reform

the Magdalene Institution following the Glasgow System that encompassed the Contagious Diseases Acts, the Lock Hospital and the Magdalene Institute. The rescue home had specific criteria for applicants since they had to be free from syphilis, could not be pregnant, had to be in the early stages of their careers as prostitutes and ready to accept strict discipline. Like in the London Lock and other English Asylums, the women were trained for a decent working-class occupation and were employed in laundry-work so that the emphasis was put on self-sacrifice, duty and repentance according to Victorian notions of class hierarchy and female inferiority and submission.[51] The same pattern of reform work clearly repeated itself throughout the century and in the various rescue institutions throughout the country.

The growing number of inmates continued to be a feature of the Lock Asylum throughout the years 1874 to 1884, just before the passing of the Criminal Law Amendment Act. Thus, 75 women were admitted in 1874 and the now existing Servants' Home provided shelter to women who had left the Asylum and sought domestic work in the capital to remain in the "paths of virtue", but who currently had nowhere else to go; in 1877, 113 women were accepted as Penitents and 91 entered the Servants' Home, and in 1879 the Asylum accepted 107 women while the Servants' Home received 36 former Penitents. Another interesting change concerning these years was that a considerable number of former inmates of the Asylum spent their holidays on the premises, and others kept in touch with the Institution through letters and visits to the Matron. During these years, there is no allusion to dismissals for elopement or negative behaviour, although these remained a constant feature of these places of confinement throughout the Victorian period.[52] Between the years 1885 and 1890 the London Lock suffered the consequences of the repeal of the Contagious Diseases Acts with a shortage of income due to the fall in legacies, annual

---

51 *Fifth Annual Report by the Directors of the Glasgow Magdalene Institution, 28 December 1864*, Special Collections Department, Glasgow University Library, accessed December 12, 2009, <http://special.lib.gla.ac.uk/exhibns/month/nov2000.html>.

52 *No 8 Annual Reports in an Octavo Bound Volume, 1873–1893* (The Library, Royal College of Surgeons of England, London), MS0022/4/2.

subscriptions and donations and to the end of the connection between the Institution and the War Office. According to the Report of 1886, "the inmates remain for a year in the Home, and during that period, they are taught to make and repair their own clothes, to wash and iron, to do general housework and plain cooking, after which they are placed out in suitable service and are provided with a complete outfit of clothes".[53] It seems that now the period of permanence had been reduced to one year. Several examples are given in the Report of former inmates who had married or established themselves in the colonies as instances of the success of the reform work done, again with a view to obtain funds at a time when there was financial trouble. Nonetheless, the number of women admitted did not decrease during these years, with 68 accepted in 1886, 88 in 1887, 72 in 1889 and 83 in 1890. In other words, the Lock Asylum, now called Rescue Home, continued to apply the same policy to the reformation of fallen women well into the last years of the century, and it looks like its income meant a significant contribution to the running of the London Lock at this stage.[54]

The Matron and the Sisters in the case of Irish Asylums or Anglican Penitentiaries were an essential part in the lives of the inmates and a point of reference for their future lives after release. At the London Lock a Matron and a Sub-matron lived in the Institution and were in charge of the women, supervising the work they did and attending to their instruction and the family worship. As we have seen in Chapter 3, Matrons had to be single mature women with firm religious beliefs; they were working-class initially, but as the century progressed they had to have an education and the proper strength to develop such difficult roles. Their salaries were low, so it was not easy to find the appropriate candidate for the job.[55] Despite all this, the Matron became like a kind of mother to the women in the Asylum, and there are many examples

---

53   *London Lock Hospital and Asylum Report 1886* (The Library, Royal College of Surgeons of England, London), MS0022/4/2.
54   *No. 8 Annual Reports in an Octavo Bound Volume, 1873–1893*, MS0022/4/2.
55   Finnegan, *Poverty and Prostitution: A Study of Victorian Prostitutes in York*, 170, 182.

The London Lock Asylum and Moral Reform 153

of the close relationship between her and some of the former inmates in the letters that they exchanged after resuming their lives outside the Asylum. In the surviving records, words of thanks like these can be frequently read:

> Dear Mrs. Hurd,
> [...] in my humble position I can only pray to God to repay you with all the blessings this world can afford for my restoration to my happy home, thereby saving me from destruction. My parents and all relatives and friends wish to convey to you and all concerned their grateful hand [sic] heartfelt thanks for kindness and care continually bestowed upon me.

> My dear Madam,
> Just a few lines to thank you all; my heart is so full I cannot express half I feel; you have been such a kind, good, dear mother to me. I know that God will reward you with a double portion of His grace. I know my dear husband is very thankful to you and dear Mr. Hurd for all your kindness to me.[56]

Mrs. Hurd was the Matron at the Lock Asylum in the 1860s and resigned in 1872, according to the records. Her husband also worked for the London Lock and she visited the women in their places of employment and wrote to them regularly after they left the Asylum. This is because the control and protection of Penitents went even beyond their release, and in the Rules for the London Lock Asylum it is established that "No inmate shall be dismissed from the Asylum after good conduct, without being provided with a respectable situation and a home".[57] They could even return if after three months they could not adapt to their new situations. Most of them were sent to service, but some were sent to the colonies where they could start a new life, to workshops or factories, or even married, and occasionally some of them died, as we can read in many of the Annual Reports of the different institutions. Their good conduct after leaving the Asylum was significantly rewarded, as the rules for the Lock Asylum establish that

---

56 *Report of the Lock Hospital and Asylum for the Years 1868, 1869, 1870, 1871*, MS0022/4/2.
57 *Laws of the London Lock Hospital and Asylum, Revised (1840)*, 1848, MS0022/5/2.

If after their restoration to society, they be found to have behaved well in their respective situations, they shall be considered as entitled to such further countenance, protection and encouragement, as the circumstances of the Institution will enable the Governors in their discretion to give.[58]

The usual reward was one guinea after twelve months in the same situation, two guineas after two years in service and three guineas if they had an adequate behaviour for three years in service in the same household.[59] It was the ladies for whom the women worked as domestic servants that sent good reports to the Institution, and here are a couple of examples:

> April, 12, 1870
> Mrs. J. wishes to express her pleasure in giving S.H. an honest and trustworthy character, as in every way deserving the present given by the Committee.
>
> November, 26, 1870
> Mrs. S. presents her compliments to Mrs. Hurd, and begs to say that S.D. has been in her service twelve months, and has conducted herself to Mrs. S.'s satisfaction in every way, and is deserving of the donation usually given.[60]

This practice was prevalent throughout the nineteenth century, but acts of rebellion and instances of bad behaviour were also quite common among these women. If one of the inmates desired to leave the Institution, she was obliged to give a month's notice, during which time the Matron and other persons in authority usually tried to convince her to stay.[61] Seclusion was voluntary, but the woman was left in isolation to think about her decision, and persuasion was employed. However, challenge to middle-class authority can be read between the lines in many of the Annual Reports and Accounts, where sentences like "requested to leave the Asylum", "received again by the Lock and other Hospitals", "eloped", "desired to leave the

---

58   *No 1, Annual Reports in an Octavo Bound Volume, 1789–1828* (The Library, Royal College of Surgeons of England, London), MS0022/4/2.
59   *An Account of the Lock Hospital; to Which is Added an Account of the Lock Asylum, 1835* (The Library, Royal College of Surgeons of England, London), MS0022/3/8.
60   *Report of the Lock Hospital and Asylum for the Years 1868, 1869, 1870, 1871*, MS0022/4/2.
61   Mahood, *The Magdalenes: Prostitution in the Nineteenth Century*, 80.

house", "dismissed for bad behaviour" or "sent to the parishes and discharged for bad conduct" can be read. Some were either transferred to other asylums or the workhouse, or sent back to the Lock or other hospitals.[62] Many of these statements probably meant the lack of success of this policy that pretended to regulate working-class women's sexual behaviour and to clean society of venereal disease and immorality. Other statements showed that many of these women became victims of syphilis again and of their recidivism in connection with their "evil courses". These were euphemisms, designed to hide the reality of reform work and are examples of resistance to power, as many Penitents did not wish to remain on the premises in spite of the attempts at persuading them, and simply left; other women were ungovernable and had an awful behaviour. They showed insolence and proved impossible for the Matrons to control. The same had also happened earlier – in, for example, the Manchester and Salford Asylum for female Penitents established in 1822, where the authorities admitted that some of the women in the Asylum had been discharged and had returned to their old ways. It was clear that the discipline and routine of confinement was very hard for some of them and were an obstacle in the moral efforts of the establishment.[63]

The inappropriate behaviour of women of the working classes was another source of concern for the people governing the Lock Asylum. In the Penitents' entries for 1824, we learn about Mary Sparks as a young woman of 18 who "is inattentive to instruction, disobedient and insolent, for which behaviour she has been put under punishment but has not yet submitted", or about Sarah Gibbon, a girl of ten who "when first received into the House possessed a perverse temper with many improper habits, some of which it is to be hoped and [sic] in a great measure eradicated". Improper habits probably meant sexual misconduct. Also Sarah Gibbs, aged 20, "possesses a sullen temper and is rather inclined to idleness than

62 *An Account of the Lock Hospital; to Which is Added an Account of the Lock Asylum, 1835*, MS0022/3/8.
63 T.J. Wyke, "The Manchester and Salford Lock Hospital, 1818–1917", *Medical History* 19, 1 (1975): 82.

industry", according to the Matron. She is also described as "very impertinent", "refractory and disobedient", and even "insolent".[64] Words like "ignorant", "insolent", "idle", "riotous" or "bad-tempered" were frequently used by the middle class to describe the lower orders of society; it can be also presumed that ignorance and rebelliousness are mentioned in these entries because they were an internal document of the institution and did not have any propagandist aim, so these appreciations must be more realistic than those found in the Accounts and Reports. The popular press and sensational newspapers similarly talked of working-class men being violent and intemperate, of women and children using bad language, and of lack of habits of personal hygiene and cleanliness in the homes.[65] By definition, such behaviour and habits had to be checked. Thus, in *The Rules for the Conduct of the Women* of the York Refuge, we find that in Rule III it is asserted that "Lying, swearing, dishonesty, repeated disobedience, and gross misbehaviour, shall be punished by the Committee with expulsion, unless circumstances should induce them to mitigate the punishment".[66] Consequently, the habits of intemperance, dishonesty or bad language typical of the working classes can probably be attributed to these women according to middle-class standards; however, it is difficult to discern to what extent these bourgeois ideas about "the poor" were not biased. It has been contended by some scholars that working-class people had their own values and behaved according to their own morality. Not all of them were so depraved, and, in fact, members of the rescue movement described some of their objects of charity and reform as the "deserving poor" but this was the prevailing image among the middle class. As a consequence of all this, silence and prayer were imposed in many of these institutions while the women were working, and lack of good conduct was punished with public reprimands, physical chastisement, isolation or even expulsion. Disruption from family and friends was also frequent to avoid bad

---

64   *Lock Asylum Committee (1836–1842)*, MS0022/2/1/4.
65   Sani D'Cruze, *Crimes of Outrage: Sex, Violence and Victorian Working Women* (London: UCL Press, 1998), 179–184.
66   Finnegan, *Poverty and Prostitution: A Study of Victorian Prostitutes in York*, 172.

influences and girls had to obtain the Matron's permission to see relatives and keep in touch with former friends.[67] Their correspondence was even supervised by the Matron both "from and to the house", according to the same York rules.

By way of conclusion, we can affirm that asylums, penitentiaries and other reform institutions for fallen women were part of a more complex structure of systems of power and gender control according to middle-class values of morality and respectability. Their success can be questioned as many of the working-class women who became inmates of these places of seclusion did not consider themselves sinners and did not comply with requirements, returning to their former habits and showing resistance to social control. Others tried to adapt to their new environments, transforming their identities and domesticating their bodies, but their voices can never be directly heard in the sources. In the case of the English institutions, most disappeared at the beginning of the twentieth century, and after World War One many of these places transformed themselves into homes for single mothers. As far as Magdalene Laundries were concerned, no records of the twentieth century have seen the light, but after 1922, with an independent Ireland, they were incorporated into the nation's architecture of containment and became more punitive and secretive in nature, with women staying longer than before. The last one closed in 1996, after being instruments of the state in the control of deviant elements of society and becoming a shameful example of female discrimination whose reverberations are still shaking Ireland's Catholic Church, well into the 21st century.

---

67 Mahood, *The Magdalenes: Prostitution in the Nineteenth Century*, 82, 89.

CHAPTER 6

The London Lock at the Turn of the Century: New Perspectives on the Physical and Moral Cure of Deviant Women

The years that elapsed between the passing of the last Contagious Diseases Act in 1869 and the repeal of regulation in 1886 brought about important changes to the London Lock. The most outstanding consequence was the eclipse of state medicine, starting in the 1870s and reaching its climax in the 1880s, which affected the state and medical control of sexuality. Throughout the repeal campaign the sanitary principle had been challenged and moralists had begun to redefine the parameters over which sexual issues were going to be discussed. With the local government reforms of the 1870s and in particular the Local Government Act of 1871, the Privy Council Medical Office and the Poor Law Board became one and formed the new Local Government Board. James Stansfeld and John Lambert became prominent figures who continued with the poor law tradition while remaining suspicious of medical experts; the latter became subordinated to civil administration, and the process culminated with Dr. Simon's resignation in 1876. The Board was more involved in the field of theoretical research on epidemics but more limited in other areas of social intervention. In other words, during the last decades of the nineteenth century sexual politics and policy were in the hands of moralists and feminists who led the way to reform through a powerful language that would oblige the state to take legislative measures. Their ideology was behind government action, and according to them "chastity, continence and self-control" were the foundation for sexual progress, and reason and the laws of human nature were essential in the process.[1]

---

1 Frank Mort, *Dangerous Sexualities: Medico-Moral Politics in England since 1830*, 2nd ed. (Routledge: London and New York, 2000), 83–87.

As stated in Chapter 4, after 1869 the numbers of patients in the London Lock Hospital decreased considerably, but still many people infected with venereal disease benefited from the Institution. The Contagious Diseases Acts were still in operation, but the *Reports* for the 1870s do not include specific information about patients, except for the number of them admitted into the Hospital and into the Asylum, and their destination once released. The knowledge we obtain from these annual statistics refers solely to the women patients at the Female Hospital in Westbourne Green and the Penitents in the Lock Asylum; there is no information about male patients in Dean Street. The figures for 1874, 1877 and 1879 are as follows:

Year	Admitted women	Admitted children/ Infants	Discharged cured	Discharged cured infants	Sent to service	Restored to friends	Sent to Lock Asylum	Sent to other Homes
1874	487 (63 married)	11	241		4	58	75	18
1877	594 (60 married)	7	294	7	4	69	113	26
1879	829 (73 married)		533			63	107	46

The first thing to attract attention in this table is the rising tendency in the number of patients admitted again throughout this decade at a time when the London Lock still counted on Government funding. Also the number of children and of married women is indicative of the presence of other individuals in the Hospital apart from prostitutes and fallen women, and is connected with the inclination to classification of inmates of different institutions that characterised the second half of the nineteenth century. Thus, in the *Report* for 1874 we can read that a re-classification of patients has been carried out "by which the respectable and least depraved women can be separated from those who have pursued an immoral career for a long period".[2] The ideology behind the call for contributions in these *Reports* is the same as in previous years: both to alleviate the consequences of the illness for "destitute fallen women" who could not resort to any other place for help, and for the blameless innocent, like infants and married women "who are compelled to seek medical advice in consequence of the immoralities of their husbands".[3] The Institution had just paid off the debts incurred because of the enlarging of buildings, but still needed the financial support of subscribers and donors. There were also Outpatients of both sexes treated at the Department in Dean Street, Soho, so monthly expenditure was growing fast in big proportions. The table also shows the destination of female patients once that had been discharged from Hospital: there were certainly many released cured, but these figures are misleading. As has been stated before, primary syphilis had visible symptoms that could disappear after treatment, but if the malady was not cured, as happened with many cases, the symptoms of secondary syphilis were not that conspicuous, which meant that the illness continued its course and spread into the population at risk. Some of those discharged were sent into service, which was the female working-class occupation par excellence, and many were restored to friends, which probably meant family and close relatives, including parents, brothers or sisters and husbands. Finally, those female patients more inclined to reform – who were more than likely the least depraved prostitutes and fallen women –, were sent either to the Lock Asylum or to other Homes, which were in most probability Magdalene Asylums, Penitentiaries or Reformatories.[4] As late as 1882, it was still believed that hardened prostitutes who were registered under the system of regulation – who represented one in seven or one in ten at that stage – hated the process and became brutalised after continuous medical inspection. They could not be reformed and were reluctant to be treated in lock hospitals; also, the women who sought for treatment

[2] *No. 8 Annual Reports in an Octavo Bound Volume*, 1873–1893 (The Library, Royal College of Surgeons of England, London), MS0022/4/2.
[3] Ibid., MS0022/4/2.
[4] *No. 8 Annual Reports in an Octavo Bound Volume*, 1873–1893, MS0022/4/2.

freely under the voluntary system at the London Lock suffered from an advanced state of the illness, making their cure almost impossible.[5]

Religious instruction was continued by Lady Visitors, City Missionaries[6] and the Chaplain in the wards, where services were held, and there were two outstanding innovations in the London Lock: the Mission Woman and the Servants' Home, which was located at Kennet Lodge in Kennet Road, St. Peter's Park. The creation of a Servants' Home was decided at a meeting of the Weekly Board on January 20th, 1876, on the initiative of Arthur Kinnaird to provide young women who had been found situations after leaving the Asylum with a temporary home when they were in periods between jobs and did not have family or friends to go to. Also some of the former inmates were allowed to spend their holidays there, always under the supervision of the Matron and the Ladies' Committee that would be in charge of this new initiative. A Ladies' Committee had been established to deal with domestic issues concerning all the branches of the Institution in 1870, which is an indication of the increasing presence of women in reform work after the Repeal Campaign.[7] Regarding the Mission Woman, she was first appointed in December 1878 in connection with the Out-patient

---

5 Edgar Beckett Truman, MD, "The Contagious Diseases Acts. To the Editor of the Lancet", *The Lancet*, November 18, 1882: 871.
6 The London City Mission was founded by a young Scottish man called David Nasmith in 1835 in the spirit of Evangelicalism. He promoted a new form of Christian ministry in the slums of big cities. He also wanted to put together the efforts of Church of England and non-conformist churches in the philanthropy work done with the poor. In the instructions for the Missionaries the ideology behind this organisation could be discerned: "Go to the people of the District assigned to you, for the purpose of bringing them to an acquaintance with salvation, through our Lord Jesus Christ, and of doing them good by every means in your power". Therefore, City Missionaries were assigned to Districts in London to teach the Gospel in increasing numbers and to instruct the working-poor in moral values that would lead them to salvation. "London City Mission", accessed August 22, 2013, <http://www.lcm.org.uk/Groups/8868/London_City_Mission/About_Us/History/History.aspx>.
7 *Patients Records, Correspondence and Plates, An Account of the Lock Hospital, from notes taken from the Minute Books* (The Library, Royal College of Surgeons of England, London), MS0022/6/3.

Clinic, at a salary of one pound per week. This new activity was known as the Dean Street Mission. According to a letter to Arthur Kinnaird from Catherine Sandars, who was in charge of the Mission in those days,

> The Mission Woman comes to the Dean Street Hospital on Fridays and Saturdays which are the days for women to attend as out-patients, and whilst the women are waiting their turn to be sent to the doctor, she engages in conversation with as many as possible, endeavours to make them feel that they have in them a friend who is ready and willing to help them, and persuades them to leave their sinful life. The other four days of the week she visits them at their homes, or rather, lodgings, because it is quite the exception for a young woman who is attending Dean Street to be living in any place that could be called a home, the majority of them living in houses kept by landladies who flourish on the sin and ruin of these young girls.[8]

As late as 1878, reformers still talk about sin and ruin to refer to prostitutes and fallen women, diverging little from the moral discourse earlier in the century. Thus the Mission Woman at the London Lock did rescue work with female out-patients, but also visited them in their places of accommodation, which were not usually a proper home as prostitutes mostly lived in lodging-houses run by working-class landladies. Missionary work became the domain of the middle-class woman in the last decades of the nineteenth century. Female philanthropists got involved in the domestic side of poverty and gave recognition to the essential role of women in the working-class family and neighbourhood. These women were free to move around the streets of London and other big cities to do their job, and exerted the power of middle-class authority over working-class households. They also controlled the resources for the poor, like housing or medical services, and on many occasions enjoyed the respect of their lower-class peers.[9] Missionary work was closely connected with the idea of social purity, which was a popular movement that tried to reach the working class through a discourse of moral reform. Militant evangelicalism was behind its pamphlets and tracts which included ideas from the Old

---

8 Ibid., MS0022/6/3.
9 Judith R. Walkowitz, City *of Dreadful Delight: Narratives of Sexual Danger in Late-Victorian London* (London: Virago Press, 1992), 55–58.

Testament about punishment and retribution for moral sinfulness. These campaigning groups tried to attract membership and personal involvement, recruiting working-class individuals who would adhere to the principles of the movement. Some of these organisations put the emphasis on preventive work and moral re-education of working-class girls and boys; also working-class mothers became the object of instruction concerning the moral education of their children and the running of their households. In the case of boys, it was important to provide them with leisure activities including sport, and night and Sunday schools to promote their education and avoid idleness.[10]

Some prominent examples of this type of organisation were the Girls' Friendly Society founded in 1874, the Ladies' Association for the Care of Friendless Girls established by Ellice Hopkins in 1876, and the Band of Hope Mission created in 1879. Ellis Hopkins (1836–1904) was an essential figure in the social purity movement and a feminist who promoted moral philanthropy among the poor. She used the language of Evangelical religion to embark on a career of public intervention to regulate morality. For her, women's physical and mental weakness was the symbol of the power of female purity, and this gave women the right to talk about sexuality, although this was a bit problematic to her as a single woman. In her view the new purity movement had to focus on two fundamental aspects: the reform of men's sexual behaviour and the implementation of moral values in the working classes, because prostitution was the consequence of male sexuality.[11] By the late 1870s, the focus of the social purity movement had moved from the repeal of the Contagious Diseases Acts to a complete transformation of society, substituting the double standard by one single standard of morality both for men and women.[12] There was a specific ideology of nationalism behind the movement, with the aim of purifying the nation and establishing the contrast with the lack of morals of

---

10   Mort, *Dangerous Sexualities: Medico-Moral Politics in England since 1830*, 88.
11   Ibid., 93–96.
12   Lesley A. Hall, *Sex, Gender, and Social Change in Britain since 1880*, 2nd ed. (London: Palgrave Macmillan, 2013), 30.

other countries. This aim was seen as above class organisation and political tendencies, and members of the middle class and the respectable working class worked together against the immorality of the aristocracy and would-be aristocrats.[13]

Prevention and education became the key words for the social purity movement. Ellice Hopkins established these two principles in the Ladies' Association for the Care and Protection of Young Girls, which had branches in many towns and cities of the United Kingdom. Their activities were based on female networking and equal rights feminism, and their charitable work was a combination of a humanitarian attitude and class pressure, in the sense that they related to the poor in a paternalist – or rather, maternalist – way. Hopkins's pamphlet *How to Start Preventive Work* outlined a structure with four aspects: an educational branch; a workhouse Magdalene branch; a preventive branch with a registry home, a free registry office and a training club; and a petitioning branch.[14]

The moral educational branch was the ideological wing of the movement and its objective was to prevent prostitution through education and to promote one single standard of morality through chastity and moderation. There were four distinct organisations, the Mothers' Union and the Women's League for married women, and the Snowdrop Bands and Evening Clubs for single young women. In the case of the first, their main preoccupation was to make mothers responsible for the education of their children, and every mother had to pledge to keep to the following guidelines:

1. To pray for the children once everyday
2. Never to allow coarse jests, bad words, or low talk before the children
3. Never to send the girls to public houses or to work at houses of bad character
4. To keep the boys and girls apart at night

---

13 Mort, *Dangerous Sexualities: Medico-Moral Politics in England since 1830*, 88–89.
14 Paula Bartley, "Preventing Prostitution: The Ladies' Association for the Care and Protection of Young Girls in Birmingham, 1887–1914", *Women's History Review* 7 (1998): 38–41.

5. To try and get the children early to bed, and not to allow our girls to keep late hours in the street
6. Never to speak of sin as a misfortune
7. To try and train the children to be truthful, honest, obedient and pure.[15]

Again, notions of working-class life can be discerned in these rules that associate poor people's behaviour with bad language, overcrowding, promiscuity, lack of religious instruction, and disorderly life. The middle-class values of honesty and purity need to be promoted among the children of the poor; keeping control over girls becomes fundamental, as it is young women who can be trained in sexual restraint, not men. At ordinary meetings of the Mothers' Union and the Women's League, subjects such as dressmaking, childcare, thrift and household economy were taught under the direction of middle-class ladies. In the case of Snowdrop Bands and Evening Clubs the target was the education of working-class girls above 11, who were instructed in honesty, chastity and civility. Their emblem was a Snowdrop as a symbol of purity.[16] On the other hand, Evening Clubs tried to make leisure activities available for young working-class girls such as needlework, singing, and quiet games. Nonetheless, all these efforts often met rejection and opposition of these working-class girls, whose class values and ways of thinking were not taken into consideration.[17]

The workhouse Magdalene branch was created to help young single women in their first illegitimate confinement to provide them with a better shelter than the city workhouse. There was a firm belief that single motherhood was the first step to prostitution, and to middle-class observers, pregnancy in women outside marriage was the living image of female sexuality. Young mothers were encouraged to find jobs in domestic service to keep their children, and they received a weekly allowance to help them with that.

---

15   Paula Bartley, *Prostitution: Prevention and Reform in England, 1860–1914* (London: Routledge, 2000), 79.
16   Bartley, "Preventing Prostitution: The Ladies' Association for the Care and Protection of Young Girls in Birmingham, 1887–1914", 42–43.
17   Bartley, *Prostitution: Prevention and Reform in England, 1860–1914*, 80–82.

At the same time, they were encouraged to apply for affiliation summonses to force fathers to pay towards the maintenance of their illegitimate children.[18] The Preventive Branch of the Ladies' Association included training homes, registry offices and clothing clubs for domestic servants. Training homes were established for wayward and troublesome girls under 18 who had not had any sexual experience, but were living in a morally dangerous environment. Therefore, parents delegated their responsibilities to the institution where they were taught in literacy, numeracy and domesticity as well as in chastity and submissiveness. The idea was to prepare them to be domestic servants and for marriage. At the same time registry offices were opened for middle-class families to hire the girls in the Society to work in their households. Finally, clothing clubs provided these girls with appropriate clothing, but they had to pay back the cost of their outfits with their salaries.[19]

Many of the activities and ideas behind all the branches of this Association have a resonance in the processes followed in the London Lock and other nineteenth-century institutions for the poor. The petitioning branch was involved in the campaign to make Parliament pass legislation to prevent juvenile prostitution and child sexual abuse, which increasingly became two of the most serious concerns for Victorians in the last decades of the nineteenth century. Both problems were connected with notions of childhood that will be discussed later in this chapter. The success of the different branches of the movement was in reality limited; the underlying difficulty was the fact that the strategies designed to deal with these working-class girls were biased by notions of gender, age and class that were predominant in middle-class reform and rescue work. Girls were classified in terms of sexual experience and age, and the depraved were separated from the chaste because the former were seen as a threat to the latter.[20]

---

18   Bartley, "Preventing Prostitution: The Ladies' Association for the Care and Protection of Young Girls in Birmingham, 1887–1914", 44–48.
19   Bartley, *Prostitution: Prevention and Reform in England, 1860–1914*, 94–97, 102–103.
20   Louise Jackson, *Child Sexual Abuse in Victorian England* (London: Routledge, 2000), 135.

Education was the other weapon of the social purity movement to combat moral depravity among the working poor: inculcating the right attitudes. In effect, it was usually easier to teach boys than girls on sexual issues, as any theoretical explanation was seen as contaminating for the latter. Boys would exercise corrupting influences among themselves, but were advised against the perils of self-abuse. Yet, it was believed that intervention at an early stage was seen as the best time for influencing the hearts and minds of the innocent young. Girls were warned against the dangers that they could face in their lives in the future, and feminists and social purity advocates were in favour of sex education for boys and girls at an early stage accomplished by their mothers at home. In the case of boys "warnings about masturbation continued" and in the case of girls the idea of "complete sexual ignorance" was contested. Sexuality as reproduction was presented as clean and pure, and the metaphor of flowers and birds was employed to describe the sexual act as a reproductive process connected with Nature.[21]

The London Lock was involved in many of these activities and initiatives described above. Through the Lock Hospital Chapel, a number of organisations were established, and their aims and functioning are described in the *Reports* of the Charities published in the 1860s and 1870s that have survived. Thus, the Friendly Visiting Society is described as created for the Ladies to visit the poor districts and give spiritual and temporal relief to the working-class families in need; also, the London City Mission, Westbourne Green District, made visits and calls, and held meetings with the poor to read the Scriptures and pray. At the same time they assisted sick people and distributed religious tracts. To encourage habits of thrift among the working classes, the Provident Society and the Westbourne Penny Provident Bank were founded by the London Lock; the first counted on visitors who collected one penny a week and at the end of the year a bonus was added to the sum saved, so that tickets were given to the savers to pay for "provisions, fuel or clothing"; the second encouraged "provident habits" among the poorer classes and feelings of "self-effort" and

---

21   Hall, *Gender, and Social Change in Britain since 1880*, 39, 55.

"self-reliance", so that interest was allowed to deposits "remaining in the Bank more than three months".[22] To relieve the material needs of the poor of the district the Soup Kitchen was run to make gallons of soup available at half price, especially to provide families with "wholesome and nutritious" food during the winter months, and the Dorcas Society used to meet every month to provide them with good clothing below its cost price, also giving some women the chance to work.[23]

As far as education and religious instruction were concerned, the Westbourne Schools in Westbourne Park were opened in 1851 for those parents who wanted their children to have an education and could not afford it, making quarterly payments. Although their curriculum is not mentioned, pupils would probably receive basic education in literacy, numeracy and the Bible. On the other hand, St. John's Servants' School located in Great Western Road and founded in 1852 was devoted to training children of the working classes to be domestic servants and their parents had to make an annual payment according to their age. Nonetheless, both institutions depended primarily on voluntary contributions.[24] The ideology of middle-class reform work was conspicuously present in the running of these Charities, and the working classes were continuously reminded of their inferior station in society. An example of this is the segregation of working-class people during services at the Lock Chapel at different days and times from their middle-class superiors. In the same fashion, Bible classes for ladies, singing classes and services for children, and Sunday and Night Schools were run in the Chapel for the benefit of young men and women who were working during the day and during the week, as we can read in the *Reports* for 1869, 1874 and 1875.

Finally, in the *Reports of the Charities* for the middle to late 1870s, detailed information about the Mission House and the Harrow Road

---

22 *Report of the Charities and Religious Societies Connected with the Lock Hospital Chapel 1864* (The Library, Royal College of Surgeons of England, London), MS0022/4/1/3.
23 *Report of the Charities and Religious Societies Connected with the Lock Hospital Chapel 1874* (The Library, Royal College of Surgeons of England, London), MS0022/4/1/3.
24 *Report of the Charities and Religious Societies Connected with the Lock Hospital Chapel 1864*, MS0022/4/1/3.

Young Men's Society is given. Established in 1874 at 61, Amberley Road, the Mission House offered the following services and meetings:

Sunday	Bible Class for Men	3 p.m.
	Bible Class for Women	3 p.m.
	Service	7 p.m.
Monday	Servants' Free Registry	11 a.m. to 1 p.m.
	Mothers' Meeting	2.30 p.m.
	Lending Library	4 to 5 p.m.
	Men's Sick and Provident Club	8 till 9.30 p.m.
Tuesday	Children's Service	6.30 p.m.
	Men's Night School	8 till 9.30 p.m.
Wednesday	Servants' Free Registry	11 a.m. to 1 p.m.
Thursday	Service	7.30 p.m.
	Men's Night School	8 till 9.30 p.m.
Friday	Servants' Free Registry	11 a.m. to 1 p.m.
	Temperance Meeting	8 p.m.
Saturday	Devotional Meeting	5 p.m.
	Penny Bank	8 till 9 p.m.[25]

The Young Men's Society was established at 6, Sutherland Gardens "for the spiritual, intellectual and social improvement of young men", providing them with facilities such as literary and debating societies, a reading room and library, and activities like classes in drawing, Greek and short-hand, Bible readings, early devotional meetings and social meetings.[26] Some of these activities and services remind us of the Ladies' Association for the Care of Friendless Girls, especially the Servants' Free Registry and the Mothers' Meeting; also the presence of the Temperance Movement with its focus on curtailing the drinking habits of the working classes can be felt amid the endeavours of these organisations. However, recreational and religious activities represented the main concern of the Young Men's

---

25　*Report of the Charities and Religious Societies Connected with the Lock Hospital Chapel 1876* (The Library, Royal College of Surgeons of England, London), MS0022/4/1/3.

26　*Report of the Charities and Religious Societies Connected with the Lock Hospital Chapel 1877* (The Library, Royal College of Surgeons of England, London), MS0022/4/1/3.

Society, aiming their work at young men of the working classes. All these initiatives formed part of a bigger national and Evangelical project which was oriented to reform and indoctrinate people from the lower orders of society. The London Lock Hospital, Asylum and Chapel were central to all this.

Moving from prevention and education to notions of Victorian childhood, several issues come to the fore, and particularly the sexual abuse of children and the problem of white slavery, which replaced official and middle-class preoccupation with the Contagious Diseases Acts in the last decades of the nineteenth century. Children began to be seen as the future of the nation and of imperialist power, but were still defined primarily as innocent. Therefore, their protection and their right to have a proper infancy and family environment became a matter of interest for Victorian minds.[27] However, the boundaries of childhood and its significance were not clear, especially the period between infancy and adulthood, that is, adolescence. It was not until the 1890s that this period of life was discerned and defined in terms of chronological age and psychological development. Before then, childhood had been defined in connection with the individual's status in relation with other groups in society. The Evangelical idea that the child was an innocent creature was checked by the Calvinist notion of the child as a wicked creature who had to be guided into adult life. As a consequence, the two familiar notions of the angel in the house and the fallen woman had their corresponding images in the child redeemer and the wayward, evil girl. The first represented the embodiment of self-sacrifice and sexual innocence; however, it was the second that represented a threat to Victorian society.[28]

Victorians had a wide collection of euphemisms to refer to child abuse such as *moral corruption, immorality, molestation, tampering, ruining* or *outrage*. Sexual abuse was defined in court as *indecent assault*,

---

27   Alan Kidd, *State, Society and the Poor in Nineteenth-Century England* (London: Macmillan Press, 1999), 85.
28   Deborah Gorham, "The 'Maiden Tribute of Modern Babylon' Re-examined: Child Prostitution and the Idea of Childhood in Late-Victorian England", *Victorian Studies* 21, 3 (1978): 369–370.

rape, unlawful carnal knowledge or its attempt, and the ambiguities and complexities surrounding it were related to Victorian constructions of gender difference, childhood, sexuality and social class. It is important to understand that child abuse was associated with female children, the same as child prostitution, but that the sexual offences were mostly committed by men. Sexual reputation affected women and not men, and the child abuse and sexual exploitation of boys was simply ignored. It was the wrong moral environment that led to corruption and delinquency, and these were the traits of the children of the poor: in the case of girls, delinquency was identified as moral depravity and early sexual knowledge; in the case of boys, delinquency was identified as theft and other criminal activities. This had as consequence the view of the female victim of sexual abuse as problematic: girls stopped being innocent and became a potential danger to other children and the rest of respectable society, transforming themselves into unnatural deviant individuals.[29] According to middle-class reformers, the problem behind child prostitution and child abuse was their working-class surroundings which endangered the innocence of children. Girls over 12 were not under their parents' surveillance any more, as they had to earn their own wages as domestic servants, dressmakers or working in the mills. Despite this, there was a significant difference between the respectable working class who tried to conform to moral standards similar to those of the middle class, not least concerning the moral behaviour of their daughters, and the unrespectable poor. The working conditions of most of the poorest outcast children were such as to make juvenile prostitution understandable. The shortage of work for girls who had to do underpaid and unskilled jobs made their lives bleak, and probably led many of them to a promiscuous life that was apparently better than their daily routines. Nevertheless, they were described by their potential middle-class reformers as flighty and unmanageable, and lacking in self-control.[30]

29   Jackson, *Child Sexual Abuse In Victorian England*, 2–6.
30   Gorham, "The 'Maiden Tribute of Modern Babylon' Re-examined: Child Prostitution and the Idea of Childhood in Late-Victorian England", 372–375.

Behind the Victorian idea of child prostitution and child abuse was the pathologising of working-class children. The existence of child rape was a living example that poor young girls did not have protection, but at the same time they were made responsible for their own fall. The way in which court cases dealt with the problem is proof that female sexuality, disease and deviancy were one and the same thing and that male sexual prerogative continued to be upheld, reinforcing once more a double standard in sexual matters.[31] The medical and legal fields of enquiry persisted in their support of discourses of power in which a class dynamic was present and made evident the control and surveillance of deviant individuals through scientific evidence. Nowadays, this would be seen as in accordance with Pierre Bourdieu's field theory. For him, different fields of practice obtain cultural authority over various objects through processes of specialisation, as was the case with medicine and law throughout the nineteenth century.[32] At this stage, the object was female sexuality, and in particular working-class girls' sexual deviance and corruption. Child rape was considered a heinous crime, but it was difficult for medical and legal experts to prove its occurrence; issues of venereal disease, working-class living conditions, blackmail and parental ignorance were put forward to determine the child's innocence and the veracity of the accusations against male perpetrators. There was a belief concerning venereal disease that if an infected male had intercourse with a virgin, his syphilis would disappear; this was considered proof of child rape, but it was used as a defence in trials; issues of torture or even murder of little children for sexual gratification were not contemplated. In any case, if there was not any symptom of venereal infection, that was seen as evidence that no violation had happened, whereas if there was venereal infection, it was thought that the child was a prostitute and responsible for her state. Also, working-class life with its connotations of poverty and immorality for middle-class minds was seen as an excuse

---

31 Mary Spongberg, *Feminising Venereal Disease: The Body of the Prostitute in Nineteenth Century Medical Discourse* (London: Macmillan, 1997), 106.
32 Pierre Bourdieu, *Outline of a Theory Practice*, trans. R. Nice (Cambridge: Cambridge University Press, 1977), 159–171.

for the existence of incest which was associated with overcrowding; once incest had taken place, the only course of life left for these children was said to be prostitution, and with it venereal disease. Similarly, issues like the veracity of parents' accusations, especially of mothers', and the possibility of blackmail as revenge or to obtain money were present in these medical and legal processes. Sometimes vaginal abnormalities were even adduced to invalidate the child's testimony against her rapist as they were interpreted as indications of an active sexual life, endorsing the model of pathological female sexuality once more; thus, the new field of criminal physiognomy of the last decades of the nineteenth century is seen here as replacing the previous model of physical anthropology.[33]

In any case, the important thing was to discover signs of external violence on the child's body, since the child's testimony was not sufficient to convict a defendant of sexual assault. The signs of abuse and how to interpret them became the crucial area of debate in this field of legal and medical discourse during the Victorian era. Taylor's *Medical Jurisprudence* (1883) was the basis for most of the medical intervention in cases of child abuse. Gender and class conceptions influenced the practice of these doctors, whose limited knowledge about venereal disease licensed their refusal to blame discharges in children on rape.[34] For lawyers and judges, respectability was the key idea during the enquiry, both in connection with the victim and the accused. Girls should be ignorant of sexual matters. To obtain the court's sympathy, girls should be shy and miserable. In other words, to be trustworthy, they had to show the prudery and innocence that were expected of a female child. Respectability was also a key element in the defence of the male defendant. The ideal of male respectability was his role as father and household head; in contrast, the sex abuser was seen as deviant according to Victorian moral standards. Almost all the males accused of rape or sexual assault gave the excuse of being under the effects of alcohol or alleged a mental disorder to mitigate their guilt. They also

---

33 Spongberg, *Feminising Venereal Disease: The Body of the Prostitute in Nineteenth Century Medical Discourse*, 110–116, 120–123.
34 Jackson, *Child Sexual Abuse in Victorian England*, 71–75.

mentioned their role as fathers so as to plead their innocence, as well as the fact that the child had offered them her sexual services in return for money, violating all notions of female respectability.[35] Male sexual pathology was never discussed and men were under the protection of notions of biological necessity, seen as impelling them towards depraved child prostitutes.

Concern about child prostitution was not new. During the 1830s and 1840s, many doctors had revealed that some children were being admitted to hospital to be treated for venereal disease. As early as 1842, the London Society for the Protection of Females and the Prevention of Juvenile Prostitution had talked about thousands of children between 10 and 16 being treated for syphilis during these decades, and we can also find examples of this in the *Annual Reports* and *Accounts* of the Lock Hospital discussed in previous chapters. The Scottish surgeon William Tait talked about the presence of very young prostitutes on the streets, and about the existence of a traffic in white slaves, although their destination was probably London. Many reformers and many members of the social purity movement believed that the only way to stop children becoming prostitutes was to change the law relating to the age of consent. There was an attempt in late 1844 to introduce a Bill for the Effectual Suppression of Brothels and Trading in Seduction that was not very much debated in the House of Lords and failed a third reading, which betrayed the knowledge of Parliament about the trade and prostitution of English girls; there were also enquiries by the Poor Law Commission, Annual Reports of the Children's Employment Commission, and Chadwick's *Report on the Sanitary Conditions of the Labouring Population* in the 1840s that gave evidence of the immorality and prostitution of working-class children and of incest in working-class families. Similarly, an Associate Institute for Improving and Enforcing the Laws for the Protection of Women was established in 1844 and an Act to Protect Women under Twenty-one from Fraudulent Practices for Procuring their Defilement was passed in 1849, which attempted a compromise between rescue workers and politicians, but was vague and had little success, keeping the age of consent at ten as

---

35   Ibid., 91–94, 117–123.

where it had been since 1576.³⁶ According to social historian Kim Stevenson, "valid consent requires that the victim fully understands her situation and is capable of exercising a rational judgement".³⁷ Hence, the age of consent can be defined as the age when a young person is legally able to consent to have sexual intercourse with another person. During the 1850s and 1860s, the object of preoccupation was child prostitution in connection with venereal disease in the debates over regulation. At this time, another bill was passed in 1861, the Offences Against the Person Act, which effectively established the age of consent at 12. What it actually did was to protect the parents' or guardians' right to control a girl's sexuality, but it did not apply to boys. Under this legislation, a young woman with property could be prevented from marrying an inappropriate suitor until the age of 21. According to this Act, it was a felony for a man to have intercourse with a child under 10 and a misdemeanour if the child was between 10 and 12; this kind of legislation went back to the thirteenth century.³⁸

During the Repeal Campaign, the fundamental issue was the seduction of children and the spread of disease, and those against regulation saw the Contagious Diseases Acts as a system of registration which encouraged girls to enter the profession, whereas those in favour of regulation believed that syphilis could be controlled and the prostitution of children could be avoided. The implications of child prostitution were discussed at the Royal Commission Regarding the Administration and Operation of the Contagious Diseases Acts of 1871. Witnesses like William Henry Sloggett, Inspector of Certified Hospitals, and Josephine Butler and Daniel Cooper were called to share their knowledge concerning child prostitution. Sloggett was a regulationist and believed that child prostitution had diminished in the districts under the Acts, but thought that it was necessary to have legislation that would allow the police to send children under the age of

---

36 Spongberg, *Feminising Venereal Disease: The Body of the Prostitute in Nineteenth Century Medical Discourse*, 127–129.
37 Kim Stevenson, "Observations on the Law Relating to Sexual Offences: the Historic Scandal of Women's Silences", accessed July 27, 2010, <http://webjcli.ncl.ac.uk/1999/issue4/stevenson4.html>.
38 Gorham, "The 'Maiden Tribute of Modern Babylon' Re-examined: Child Prostitution and the Idea of Childhood in Late-Victorian England", 362–364.

16 to reformatories or industrial schools.[39] Mary Carpenter was the first to raise the issue of reform of the destitute child through the creation of reformatories and industrial schools in the 1850s. She attributed the depraved state of the poor young to poverty and the lack of parental love, and thought that the solution was to remove the child from that morally corrupting atmosphere.[40] The Industrial Schools Act of 1866 permitted taking children begging, wandering or destitute and in bad company, to certified industrial schools. However, it was not until 1880 that The Industrial Schools Act, also known as the Ellis Hopkins Act in recognition of her campaign, was passed. It gave local authorities the right to remove children from disorderly and immoral homes and place them in industrial schools. Cooper and Butler gave evidence reporting the bad effects of the application of the Acts as, in their opinion, registration of girls under 16 led to an increase in child prostitution, and the system hindered their escape from the profession. According to them, these children were always in the company of older prostitutes, and became brutalised and more difficult to be reformed. Cooper and Butler insisted that the situation would only improve by punishing seduction and raising the age of consent. The Majority Report recommending the continuation of the Contagious Diseases Acts has already been discussed in another chapter; however, in relation to child prostitution and child abuse, it also recommended raising the age of consent, sending girls under 16 found on the streets to industrial schools and eliminating brothels and procurers. As a result, Home Secretary Bruce tried to introduce a bill in Parliament in 1872 that would implement the suggested reforms, superseding the Acts, raising the age of consent to 14 and introducing harder penalties for procurers and brothel-keepers. His bill was thrown out. Only in 1875, did the House of Commons make amendments to the Offences Against the Person Act raising the age of consent from 12 to 13.[41]

39 Spongberg, *Feminising Venereal Disease: The Body of the Prostitute in Nineteenth Century Medical Discourse*, 132–133.
40 Kidd, *State, Society and the Poor in Nineteenth-Century England*, 87.
41 Spongberg, *Feminising Venereal Disease: The Body of the Prostitute in Nineteenth Century Medical Discourse*, 133–136.

Simultaneously, Alfred Dyer, a publisher who specialised in social purity books and pamphlets, was finding evidence of a traffic of English girls to the Continent. He demonstrated that the trade was taking place in countries like Belgium, France and Holland when he travelled to Belgium himself and found English girls in licensed brothels. They were obliged to contract a debt with the brothel-owners which kept them prisoners. After organising popular agitation against the situation, the London Committee for the Suppression of the Traffic in British Girls for the Purposes of Continental Prostitution was created with the support of Benjamin Scott, Chamberlain of the City of London, and former prominent members of the Repeal Campaign such as Josephine Butler, William Shaen and Henry Wilson. In addition, the Home Office had appointed barrister Thomas Snagge to carry out an investigation to prove that English girls had been abducted to continental brothels. He obtained absolute certainty that the facts were happening and gave detailed information about women being inscribed on police registers as prostitutes in continental brothels. These houses of ill fame were controlled by a special police of morals which was corrupt and repressive at the same time. He also proved that English law and administration had loopholes that permitted the transaction.[42]

In 1880, Josephine Butler published a letter in the *Shield* entitled "The Modern Slave Trade" which did not bring much expectation in England but attracted Belgian authorities who asked her to share her knowledge with a magistrate, so "she sent a sworn deposition to the Home Office".[43] Private prosecution took place against Belgian brothel-keepers and four prostitute girls under twenty-one gave evidence of their having been kidnapped and treated in a brutal way. These British girls were rescued by Alfred Dyer, a young Quaker missionary, but the results of the trial caused some uproar in England. A Select Committee was established in 1881 to make a reluctant Parliament consider the investigation of the Traffic of English Girls

---

42 Gorham, "The 'Maiden Tribute of Modern Babylon' Re-examined: Child Prostitution and the Idea of Childhood in Late-Victorian England", 357–360.
43 Spongberg, *Feminising Venereal Disease: The Body of the Prostitute in Nineteenth Century Medical Discourse*, 137–138.

to Foreign Destinations. The Committee concluded that police methods were ineffective in preventing child prostitution in London and the spread of venereal disease in children. It also considered the information given by Snagge on the slave trade and produced a report. Some witnesses maintained that seduction and poverty were the main causes of juvenile prostitution, but others gave evidence as to the presence of working-class girls on the streets who manipulated the sexual and economic opportunities available with the police and their potential clients-seducers.[44] Members of Parliament and the upper classes opposed legislative reform because they believed that prostitution was necessary and unavoidable and they felt themselves and their sons would be threatened by those measures. Many police inspectors denied the existence of a white slave trade, and many believed that it was just simply un-British to let it flourish on English soil. They even alleged that prostitutes chose their own fate and thought that women who had lost all trace of chastity had no redeeming values.[45]

On the other hand, social purists wished to protect young women from the sexual exploitation of older men. In other words, they wanted to extend the protection that middle-class girls enjoyed to the daughters of the working class and to give them shelter without taking into consideration their circumstances and ways of thinking.[46] In this sense, the rhetoric of the white slavery metaphor became instrumental, because it redefined the figure of the prostitute as the victim of social and economic devices that were beyond her control. Censure was redirected from the victim to the exploiter, from the individual to society, and from women to men. The image of the black slave in abolitionist ideology was substituted by the demoralised white woman whose sexual labour was even more abhorrent than slavery itself. This encouraged repealers and new abolitionists to pool efforts in the anti-regulation campaign.[47] However, it was not until

44 Ibid., 138–140.
45 Mary Ann Irwin, *"White Slavery" As Metaphor Anatomy of Moral Panic*, <http://userwww.sfsu.edu/epf/journal_archive/volume_V,_1996/irwin_m.pdf>, accessed August 23, 2013.
46 Hall, *Sex, Gender, and Social Change in Britain since 1880*, 33.
47 Irwin, *"White Slavery" As Metaphor Anatomy of Moral Panic*.

W.T. Stead published his series of articles entitled "The Maiden Tribute of Modern Babylon" in the *Pall Mall Gazette* in the summer of 1885 and the public uproar it provoked that Parliament passed legislation to protect women and children from white slavery and sexual exploitation.

Using the techniques of new journalism such as melodrama and the universal interview – a form of direct interview that gave voice to a considerable number of women –, Stead acquainted a middle- and working-class readership with the stories of young girls who had been victims of seduction. Sensationalist stories were filling the pages of the yellow press in the last decades of the nineteenth century and sexual crimes figured prominently in them.[48] Similarly, melodrama was another popular genre, especially among the lower orders of society, and particularly domestic melodrama referred to the upper-class male villain, along with a passive plebeian hero and a passive female victim who was the heroine.[49] It was the combination of all these elements that made Stead's stories a great success. According to him, a "Secret Commission" was established to explore the London underworld and obtain evidence about the violation of virgins and the existence of a white-slave trade. His main objective was to make Parliament consider passing legislation that would protect English women and children from prostitution and white slavery. He described how innocent girls were taken to London and were given drinks and drugs to be raped by men who would pay a considerable amount of money for their virginity. They were working-class girls who were orphans or daughters of drunken parents who sold them to procurers; once they were corrupted they remained in the streets as prostitutes.[50] Stead also demonstrated the existence of a slave traffic in both directions between England and the continent, with girls coming from France, Belgium, Germany and Switzerland

---

48   Shani D'Cruze, *Crimes of Outrage: Sex, Violence and Victorian Working Women* (London: UCL Press, 1998), 77.
49   Walkowitz, *City of Dreadful Delight: Narratives of Sexual Danger in Late-Victorian London*, 86.
50   W.T. Stead, "The Maiden Tribute of Modern Babylon", *Pall Mall Gazette*, July 6, 1885 (The Women's Library, London Metropolitan University), 3/AMS/B/01/01-04, Box 36.

to work in London brothels, and English women and girls travelling to the continent for the purposes of sexual exploitation. He insisted on the innocence and poor conditions of the victims and considered them too young to be conscious of the decisions they were taking.[51] He even took part in one of the transactions with a girl named Elizabeth Armstrong which brought very serious consequences for him and for those who had helped him in the process, the midwife who certified the little girl's virginity, Mme. Mourez, and the procuress Rebecca Jarrett.[52]

Since at least the late 18th century, stories of seduction of a working-class girl by a profligate aristocrat had proliferated. Now the confrontation between social classes contributed to the transformation of the white-slavery metaphor into a full-blown moral panic. The fact that Stead had staged the problem in London was a decisive factor together with the impact of a potent newspaper with mass circulation in the rest of the country.[53] Those who opposed the new measures argued that they represented a threat to personal liberty and that the powers of the police would be once more enlarged to control public space and individuals. They did not want the state to regulate sexuality. They preferred a system of voluntary surveillance and control by private individuals through voluntary rescue work. Nonetheless, support was achieved in the end from clergymen, Liberals, social purists, trade-union leaders and feminists, and the way in which Stead presented the drama of sexual exploitation made participants in the agitation forget their conflicts and contradictions and their class and political implications.[54] After the articles were published hundreds of letters were

---

51 W.T. Stead, "The Maiden Tribute of Modern Babylon", *Pall Mall Gazette*, July 10, 1885 (The Women's Library, London Metropolitan University), 3/AMS/B/01/01-04, Box 36.

52 For a detailed description and interpretation of Stead's series of articles on "The Maiden Tribute of Modern Babylon", see M.I. Romero Ruiz, "Women's Identity and Migration: Stead's Articles in the *Pall Mall Gazette* on Prostitution and White Slavery" in *Cultural Migrations and Gendered Subjects: Colonial and Postcolonial Representations of the Female Body*, ed. Silvia P. Castro Borrego and Maria Isabel Romero Ruiz (Newcastle-upon-Tyne: Cambridge Scholars Publishing, 2011), 27–53.

53 Irwin, *"White Slavery" As Metaphor Anatomy of Moral Panic.*

54 Mort, *Dangerous Sexualities: Medico-Moral Politics in England since 1830*, 81, 100–101.

sent by statesmen, clergymen, housewives and all kinds of people to the *Pall Mall Gazette* and other provincial and national newspapers supporting the passing of the proposed bill to raise the age of consent. This bill had passed the House of Lords in 1883, but had failed to pass the House of Commons several times between 1883 and 1885; several large public meetings had taken place in the Exeter Hall and the Princess Hall in London, and Josephine Butler and Ellice Hopkins were among the leaders. Also, a petition with 393,000 signatures had been presented to the Government by the Salvation Army to increase pressure to enforce the new legislation, and on 7 August 1885, the Bill was passed after a third reading, becoming law a week later.[55] Its complete title was "An Act to make further provision for the Protection of Women and Girls, the suppression of brothels, and other purposes", and it was full of significance. A few days later, on 22 August, a huge meeting was held at St. James's Hall where the National Vigilance Association was formed, whose aim was to protect young girls and to ensure the application of the new Criminal Law Amendment Act of 1885. It was also the aim of this social purity organisation to combat juvenile prostitution and the traffic in girls and women. In 1899, it institutionalised its international dimension with the foundation of the International Bureau for the Suppression of the Traffic in Persons in 1899.[56]

With the Criminal Law Amendment Act the procuration of a woman or girl for the purposes of prostitution in a British or a European brothel was regarded as a crime; carnal knowledge of a girl under 13 was considered a felony; and sexual assault on a girl between 13 and 16 or on an imbecile woman was seen as a misdemeanour. Penalties oscillated between two years and penal servitude, and it was explicitly mentioned that no woman could be forced to have sexual intercourse by the use of drugs or any other substance. Brothel-owners could similarly be convicted and be fined or sent to prison. Homosexuality was regulated for the first time in the history of sexuality as sodomy and defined as gross indecency in Section 12; it was

---

55 Irwin, *"White Slavery" As Metaphor Anatomy of Moral Panic*.
56 Gorham, "The 'Maiden Tribute of Modern Babylon' Re-examined: Child Prostitution and the Idea of Childhood in Late-Victorian England", 361–362.

regarded as a misdemeanour liable to conviction, and it remained as such till 1967.[57] Section 4 contemplated the possibility of the testimony of a child, not on oath and if the Court agreed to it, which represented an important step for the work done by the Society for the Prevention of Cruelty to Children (SPCC). This Society devoted its efforts to investigating and bringing to trial cases of child abuse and neglect. Now a warrant could be issued to remove girls or women from places where they were detained against their wills for immoral purposes and to take them back to their parents or guardians.[58] The SPCC functioned as a body of professional inspectors following a straightforward policy based on a systematic programme of welfare intervention which amounted to regular visits, advice and warning, normally focused on working-class homes. Legal advice was also given, since the number of prosecutions grew considerably after 1885.[59] In this respect the Industrial Schools Act of 1880 was crucial, in that it allowed local authorities to remove children from disorderly and immoral homes and place them in Industrial Schools. Nonetheless, it was not until a series of acts such as the Protection of Children Act of 1889, the Custody of Children Act of 1891 and the Punishment of Incest Act of 1908 that judges were allowed to take the custody of children from parents in situations of neglect and ill-treatment and that incest was made a secular crime.

The National Vigilance Association (NVA) was then born out of a previous organisation, the Society for the Suppression of Vice, which had been established in 1802 to fight pornography, and began with this Society's account's balance, although it had a broader scope. Women and workers were among its members, but it was predominantly a middle-class organisation with a feminist stamp.[60] The NVA feminists' objective was the purification

---

57 *Criminal Law Amendment Act, 1885 (An Abstract)* (The Women's Library, London Metropolitan University), 3/AMS/B/01/01-04, Box 36.
58 Jennifer Payne, "The Criminal Law Amendment Act of 1885 and Sexual Assault on Minors", accessed September 13, 2009.,<http://www.geocities.com/Athens/Aegean/7023/Consent.html>.
59 Jackson, *Child Sexual Abuse in Victorian England*, 52, 64–65.
60 Celia Marshik, *British Modernism and Censorship* (Cambridge: Cambridge University Press, 2006), 2.

and civilisation of the public and private worlds because of the fear of a working-class uprising. The 1880s were a period of economic and political instability with the development of socialism, a big growth of trade unionism and an increase in foreign migration to the East End of London. These changes led to a reconfiguration of the working classes, plus a wider appropriation of middle-class concepts of respectability. At the same time, the undeserving poor became the dangerous class which had to be monitored and repressed to keep social order. These feminists were influenced by religious beliefs and endorsed the temperance movement, viewing poor women as victims of male alcoholics.[61] The Association had its own journal, *The Vigilance Record*, and its main aims were the reform of male sexuality and a coercive policy of sexual regulation through the fight against pornography, various forms of public entertainment, and the control of sexual practices like incest, masturbation and contraception – all seen as immoral.[62] Under the leadership of William Coote, the National Vigilance Association took measures that were simultaneously progressive and regressive, liberal and conservative. For example, at the executive meeting of 1886 several issues were considered to form part of their agenda: the danger of local resistance to the repeal campaign, the problem of men soliciting women, preventive education work, information about local refuges, Italian organ-grinders, rowdyism in the streets, immorality in parks, theatre children, the plea of "reasonable belief" that the girl was 16 in abuse cases, the possibility for women of having female friends with them in court cases, and the introduction into law of several new sexual offences.[63]

Prostitution was still a preoccupation, although the National Vigilance Association directed its attention to the partially fallen and the younger prostitute, ignoring the hardened prostitute who still found social hostility and stigmatisation. Josephine Butler began to deplore the repressive nature of the Association, as did other feminists who had belonged to the Ladies'

---

61   Lucy Bland, "'Purifying' the Public World: Feminist Vigilantes in Late Victorian England", *Women History Review* 1, 3 (1992): 398–399.
62   Judith R. Walkowitz, "Male Vice and Female Virtue: Feminism and the Politics of Prostitution in Nineteenth Century Britain", *History Workshop Journal* 13 (1982): 84.
63   Hall, Lesley *Sex, Gender, and Social Change in Britain since 1880*, 38.

National Association like Elizabeth Wolstenholme Elmy, especially in connection with the clauses in the Criminal Law Amendment Act related to brothels. Under this, landlords were made responsible for letting property to suspected prostitutes to pursue their business, which meant that many would not hire rooms to them. This created a housing problem, not only for prostitutes, but also for women living with other women or living on their own. Therefore, women turned to the streets and to setting up house with pimps to obtain protection and cover for their work, changing the tendency of the previous years when prostitution had been a female business.[64]

Regarding pornography, the National Vigilance Association focused its attention on obscene publications, which, as stated in Chapter 4, had remained a middle- and upper-class business for the literate and educated until late in the century. However, in the 1880s and 1890s, pornography was becoming more accessible through the development of photography and the pornographic postcard. The latter was cheap to produce and reached the working classes, dealing with topics that had subversive connotations, but which also catered to new tastes with the addition of exotic and Oriental elements. Similarly women appeared in them surrounded by a natural world of flowers and animals. The Association pressured New Scotland Yard to create a special department for prosecuting indecent books and pictures. As far as contraception was concerned, birth-control was still viewed as connected with illicit and promiscuous sex.[65]

Another important issue for the executive committee was the protection of children and girls from sexual abuse. Between 1890 and 1910 a compromise between state and various organisations was behind most prosecutions, many of which were initiated by the National Vigilance Association which devoted half of its annual budget to these legal processes. At the same time, a new cooperation was born between the Association and the police that counted on some members to combat child abuse. In this, purity groups and the police exchanged information and worked

---

64 Bland, "'Purifying' the Public World: Feminist Vigilantes in Late Victorian England", 400–401.
65 Hall, *Sex, Gender, and Social Change in Britain since 1880*, 38–40, 56.

together in cases related to brothels, obscenity and abduction. In this sense, the Association had also a prominent role in denouncing cases of incest and promoting legislation to put an end to this.[66] Incest was identified as a working-class problem due to overcrowding, as noted, but working-class women and men were encouraged to participate in this coercive policy through surveillance of their children's sexuality. Working-class mothers were given the moral authority to teach their girls sexual respectability, but these young women could not have a future free from a hard life without any hope for improvement. The assumption was that they did not know about sexual matters and could not control their bodies for reproduction. In the same vein, boys and young men should not indulge in self-abuse and sexual intercourse. Similarly, working-class fathers were expected to become responsible patriarchs who abided by the same domestic ideology.[67]

Finally, the music-hall and other public spectacles became the target of the National Vigilance Association, in a struggle to preserve decency. Music-halls flourished in the last decades of the nineteenth century, emerging as a form of working-class culture. Women could be found in the audience, and prostitutes resorted to these places to meet clients. The idea was to eliminate vice and alcohol from music-halls and transform them into respectable family entertainment through the inspection by purity workers collaborating with the London City Council.[68] Feminists were thus concerned with making the public arena a safe place for decent women to move about town without the fear of being molested or identified as prostitutes, thus purifying the world outside the home.

In the years between the passing of the Criminal Law Amendment Act and the end of the Victorian era, the London Lock suffered the consequences of the repeal of the Contagious Diseases Acts, especially in the lack of state funding and a lack of medical innovation as far as treatment and advances of medicine were concerned. The London Lock showed little

---

66 Mort, *Dangerous Sexualities: Medico-Moral Politics in England since 1830*, 104–105.
67 Walkowitz, "Male Vice and Female Virtue: Feminism and the Politics of Prostitution in Nineteenth Century Britain", 85.
68 Lucy Bland, *Banishing the Beast: Feminism, Sex and Morality* (London and New York: Tauris Parke Paperbacks, 2002), 118.

activity and progress till after the First World War and the establishment of the Royal Commission on Venereal Disease in 1917. In this period, venereology and dermatology came quite close and ophthalmology made a significant contribution to the treatment of eye complaints derived from venereal disease and of ophthalmia neonatorum, which affected infants who got infected from their mothers with gonococcal vaginal discharges at childbirth. At the same time, mercury was gradually being replaced by other alternative treatments, but it was not until the discovery of salvarsan that sexually transmitted diseases could be controlled by the use of chemical substances. The staff at the London Lock was made of competent but traditional medical practitioners who practised in the conventional way of the time without the stimulus of academic research. Venereology was not a recognised medical speciality in the United Kingdom and, in general hospitals, cases of secondary and tertiary syphilis were treated by physicians specialising in dermatology, male patients with primary chancre or gonorrhoea were treated by surgeons, and female patients with gonorrhoea were treated by gynaecologists. Women with syphilis were transferred to general physicians or to the London Lock, whereas patients with tabes dorsalis or general paralysis were sent to workhouses and lunatic asylums. In the case of the London Lock Hospital, all patients were under the treatment of surgeons who had to be certified members of the Royal College of Surgeons of England and usually had other appointments in other hospitals, although the tendency in these years was to work on venereal disease alone. However, at this stage, the Zittman method, which consisted in treating a patient with tertiary syphilis by keeping them in a very hot room to provoke an abundant sweat with large doses of sarsaparilla, was used together with potassium iodide which made it a slightly more effective treatment. Operations continued to be carried out at the London Lock, and plastic surgery became prominent; this meant the need of an anaesthetic and a pathological laboratory. Medical students were allowed to see patients at the male department but not at the Female Hospital.[69]

---

69   David Innes Williams, *The London Lock: A Charitable Hospital for Venereal Disease, 1746–1952* (London and New York: Royal Society of Medicine Press Ltd., 1995), 99–106.

The numbers of patients admitted into the Female Hospital were still very high: 546 during 1886, 642 during 1888 and 731 during 1890, but the main problem was funding. In the *Report* for 1886, the Weekly Board of Governors complains of the serious falling off in donations and annual subscriptions. They also appeal to those who stopped giving support because of the application of the Contagious Diseases Acts: repeal of those Acts had brought an end to Government funding. The resulting shortage of funds, they say, had occasioned the closure of thirty beds and had forced the rejection of many applications for admission. Similarly, and due to the situation, it was decided that the different Reformatory Homes and Refuges which, till then, had sent patients to the Female Hospital without making any contribution to their maintenance would be charged 6 shillings per week from 1 January 1887. In the text, potential contributors are reminded that "fifty pounds in one payment or in two payments within two years constitutes a Life Governor, and five guineas annually an annual Governor".[70]

The West Wing or the Duke of Cambridge Wing was devoted to the Asylum, now called Rescue Home, and a Library for the use of patients and nurses was opened. The Report blames false delicacy among potential donors as one reason for the decline in contributions: false, not least because the number of people affected by the disease had not diminished at all. As a way of propaganda and to obtain extra money, illustrated booklets entitled "Upward Steps in Rescue Work" describing the Hospital and Asylum were published and sold; also from the year 1890 onwards pictures of the buildings outside and inside where inmates and patients could be seen in their daily routine were found in the *Reports*. These signify a clear indication of the advantages of the use of photography in rescue and philanthropy work by the end of the century.[71]

Regarding the nursing and administration of the Hospital, in the 1890s matrons tried to retrain nurses working at the London Lock to

---

70 *London Lock Hospital and Asylum Report 1886* (The Library, Royal College of Surgeons of England, London), MS0022/4/2.
71 *London Lock Hospital and Asylum Report 1891* (The Library, Royal College of Surgeons of England, London), MS0022/4/2.

cover attendance of more than one hundred beds. Three certified nurses and nine probationers were hired for a course that lasted two years, after which they could work either in the Asylum or in another hospital. They were provided with accommodation in a nurses' home but it was difficult to recruit them because of the nature of the illness and because they could not obtain a national certificate after training at the London Lock. Male nurses attended male patients at Dean Street. In 1891, a registrar without a salary was appointed as a junior officer to keep the records, and the Secretary was now in charge of the two hospitals and lived in a house in Harrow Road. A Medical Committee was established and the Ladies' Committee now extended their influence to the Hospital, following the late-19th-century trend of an increasing presence of women in philanthropy work and the public sphere.[72] The number of Surgeons and other junior medical officers was also increased, owing to the growing number of out-patients at the Dean Street Hospital. The Board decided that male out-patients could be seen two evenings a week and on Saturday afternoons, as many of them could not attend during the day because of pressure of work. As a consequence, the number of male out-patients increased by more than fifty per cent, and female out-patients that had been treated in the Female Hospital were allowed to continue their treatments one afternoon a week. In all probability, this meant a further burden on the finances of the Hospital. Another important decision was also taken in these years in relation to the Lock Chapel as its management and maintenance were going to be in the hands of the Chapel Congregation. The latter was represented through its Committee and by the Chaplain, who would have free use of the Lock Parsonage. The Chaplain would continue doing the same duties – visiting patients in the wards once a week, instructing the girls in the Rescue Home and chairing the Ladies' Committee –, although he did not have to lend his services to the Hospital in Dean Street.[73]

72 Innes Williams, *The London Lock: A Charitable Hospital for Venereal Disease, 1746–1952*, 107–109.
73 *London Lock Hospital and Asylum Report 1888* (The Library, Royal College of Surgeons of England, London), MS0022/4/2.

By the end of the nineteenth century, many lock hospitals and lock wards in general hospitals were being closed, and Infirmary lock wards were malfunctioning. According to the testimony of a doctor who had visited one of the Poor-law lock words in 1900 and had been himself in charge of one of them, the food and treatment in Infirmaries was not good, and nurses were insufficiently trained; hygienic conditions were deplorable as well, making patients leave the institution before they had been cured.[74] However, even more worrying was the fact that some lock hospitals were being closed, like the Liverpool Lock Hospital, and the number of beds in lock wards of general hospitals was being alarmingly reduced, especially in London. The Liverpool Lock Hospital catered for patients from the merchant marine and Royal Navy, and had a prestigious medical school, but its closure was attributed to the persisting stigma of venereal disease. Ignorance and lack of prevention were still behind the spread of the malady.[75] Lack of funding was the cause for the reduction in the number of facilities and beds, but men, women and children with syphilis continued deserving charity and treatment. At the same time the incidence of venereal disease was not diminishing in frequency or severity, and it was becoming even more virulent in certain areas than in previous years. Ideas about treating the disease independently from the way it had been contracted began to emerge, making a new conception of medicine possible.[76] Although the London Lock Hospital in Dean Street was attended by a considerable number of out-patients, many of them still needed treatment as in-patients. Medical students also needed to obtain experience from hospital practice, as big cities like London and small towns needed lock hospitals and lock wards.[77]

---

74   M.D. Lond, D.P.H. Cantab., "Treatment in Infirmary Lock Wards", *The British Medical Journal*, November 24, 1900: 1537.
75   S.J. Ross, "The Liverpool Lock Hospital. To the Editors of *The Lancet*", *The Lancet*, April 22, 1899: 1120.
76   "Reminiscences of the Liverpool Lock Hospital", *The Lancet*, February 2, 1907: 305–306.
77   Frederick W. Lowndes, "Lock Hospitals and Lock Wards. To the Editors of *The Lancet*", *The Lancet*, April 1, 1899: 927.

The main problem was a range of factors which boosted the cost of voluntary hospitals and hospitals in general. New treatments required more advanced equipment, the creation of special departments, the enlargement of medical staff, and the more frequent practice of surgery implied the necessity to control hospital infections with the increase of expenses associated with the improvement of hygiene and the use of antiseptics. In the same manner, improving the quality of nursing signified increased costs and providing nurses with in-house accommodation, and sometimes re-building and refurbishment were necessary, which meant extra expenditure. Popular perception of hospital care was changing with associations of good nursing, and there was a massive increase in the number of in-patients and out-patients that resorted to medical facilities and services. At the same time, by the 1870s, increasing concern connected with the abuse of charitable hospital facilities was becoming common among those people influenced by the ideology of self-help.[78] Consequently, new ways were needed for fund-raising and to cover expenses for medical assistance. Organisations such as the Charity Organisation Society and the British Hospitals Association were involved in obtaining financial support and detecting financial irregularities and shortages in voluntary hospital provision. Thus, donations and legacies continued to be an important source of income, and the rent or sale of plots of land began to be a common practice to secure an extra source of money for long established institutions. For example, at the London Lock, a Special Board of July 1886 decided to sell a plot of land to the Board of Guardians of Paddington for the sum of 2,000 pounds, as the cumulative debt had now reached £4,500. The Annual Dinner of 1889 brought an extra sum of 2050 pounds, and the Kinnaird Memorial Fund another 553 pounds. Annual dinners were another form of raising money for voluntary hospitals, and in 1890 it was confirmed that the Asylum with its laundry and other work and the Out-patients Department with patients' fees were contributing an income of 1,000 pounds annually each.

---

78 Steven Cherry, "Hospital Sunday, Workplace Collections, and Issues in Late Nineteenth-Century Hospital Funding", *Medical History* 44 (2000): 461, 465–467.

But the Female Hospital represented a heavy burden on the finances of the Institution.[79] To control the financial situation, several measures were proposed by the Secretary, Mr. A.W. Cruikshank, who now made a report where he included six recommendations:

1. To make appeals for the Hospital and Rescue Home separately.
2. To invite subscriptions from the residents of Paddington through the Church congregational Collectors.
3. Send out appeals.
4. Advertise.
5. Hold a bazaar in tents in the grounds as well as the dinner.
6. The office of collector, which had lapsed in 1875, should be revived.

The last proposed measure had to do with the fall in annual subscriptions and contributions which had been an important source of income in the eighteenth century and earlier in the nineteenth. With all these steps, the debt was reduced to less than a hundred pounds in 1897, but by the turn of the century it had already grown to 3,000 pounds again.[80] The old system of Governors who could recommend admissions had completely disappeared, and now patients were only accepted on medical recommendation and the Annual General Meeting was now open to the public. As a result, being a Governor was just an honorific position with no power to take decisions regarding patients or to influence Hospital policy. This would explain the reduction in the number of subscriptions.

Other methods of obtaining funds were the Hospital Sunday, the Hospital Saturday, and the works collections. The Hospital Sunday was an annual Sunday event when collections in all the churches took place through an appeal sermon which went to a central fund; then the money obtained would be distributed among the hospitals in need. Hospital Saturday consisted of street collections, donations and fund-raising by Friendly Societies,

---

79 *Patients Records, Correspondence and Plates, An Account of the Lock Hospital, from notes taken from the Minute Books*, MS0022/6/3.
80 Ibid., MS0022/6/3.

and workplace collections meant workers' payments through sick clubs or other methods. One problematic aspect of the latter, though, was that worker-contributors began to claim a right to access hospital care and even to take part in hospital government.[81] But the organisation that lasted longer and was more influential was the Prince of Wales Hospital Fund for London, which was formed in 1897. It encompassed donations from companies and philanthropists who desired to count on the King's favour, comprising a big endowment fund which was to support the London voluntary hospitals. At the same time, it would exert some kind of control over hospital management till the creation of the National Health Service, and changed its name to the King's Fund in 1901.[82] The London Lock certainly benefited from all these forms of fund raising.

In the aftermath of the Criminal Law Amendment Act positive and negative implications could be discerned. The truth was that the new legislation accomplished very little and in some instances worked against feminist goals, because it emphasised the idea of women's helplessness, undermining claims to social, economic and legal equality with men. Also, the attempts to succeed in the generalisation of a single moral standard led to an increase in repressive measures directed at women, which involved an attack on libertarian attitudes via an interference in private sexuality. But all the while a cross-class alliance between women developed, together with a more open discussion of women's sexual practices, which gradually allowed women to have control and autonomy over their bodies.[83] One of the most prominent new features of the last decades of the nineteenth century was the emergence of sexology with its consequences for homosexuality and the history of sexuality in general, with Havelock Ellis as an outstanding figure in the discipline.

As stated above, in the Criminal Law Amendment Act of 1885, homosexuality described as sodomy was criminalised both in public and

---

81 Cherry, "Hospital Sunday, Workplace Collections, and Issues in Late Nineteenth-Century Hospital Funding", 740–471, 482–483.
82 Innes Williams, *The London Lock: A Charitable Hospital for Venereal Disease, 1746–1952*, 111–112.
83 Irwin, *"White Slavery" As Metaphor Anatomy of Moral Panic*.

in private for the first time in English history. The clause was known as the Labouchère amendment, and there was no age limit; it was defined as "gross indecency" and categorised as "indecent assault", that is, it was seen a lesser offence treated in a similar way to infanticide as it did not require medical evidence. It seems that the Act originally contained an allusion to same-sex between women, but Queen Victoria herself rejected it because for her the existence of an offence in women comparable to buggery was inconceivable. So lesbianism was not classified as a crime.[84] Nonetheless, with the advances in the studies of sex, there was a common development in continental and English medical and legal discourses. They moved from the description of physical signs of sodomy – following again Taylor's *Medical Jurisprudence* (1883) where sodomy was defined as "the unnatural connection of a man with a man" – to the new concept of the "pervert" or "homosexual type". The development of sex psychology allowed doctors and other specialists to talk about sex outside venereology and forensic medicine.[85] Thus, the emergence of sexology in Britain under the influence of the advances and new theories in North-America and the continent took place in the late 1880s and 1890s. Sexology has been seen as reaction to the monolithic system of Victorian repression on the one hand and as a new attempt to control the individual's sexuality with the creation of the "pervert" on the other hand. In any case, sexual science is indebted to feminism and the social purity movement, because they brought to public debate issues of moral and sexual behaviour and questioned assumptions about what was normal or natural in relation to male and female sexuality.[86]

Several publications contributed to the construction of the new science. Patrick Geddes and J. Arthur Thomson's *The Evolution of Sex* was published in 1889, a cheap volume that circulated widely and viewed human sexuality as linked to reproduction. According to them, males and females

---

84 Hall, *Sex, Gender, and Social Change in Britain since 1880*, 34–35.
85 Ivan Dalley Crozier, "The Medical Construction of Homosexuality and its Relation to the Law in Nineteenth-Century England", *Medical History* 45 (2001): 62–63.
86 Lesley A. Hall, "Hauling Down the Double Standard: Feminism, Social Purity and Sexual Science in Late Nineteenth Century Britain", *Gender and History* 16, 1 (2004): 37–38, 43.

were complementary but Geddes and Thompson had an ambivalent stance towards artificial birth-control and advocated temperance. For his part, Edward Carpenter who was a mystical social reformer, endorsed a celebratory position in relation to the body and promoted a relationship between the sexes close to comradeship. He first published a series of pamphlets on questions of sex reform, but these formed the basis for his book *Love's Coming of Age* of 1896, although his section on "The Intermediate Sex" did not appear until 1906. He believed in the biological differentiation of the sexes but considered excessive the social differences between them. Carpenter saw sex as a union and assigned women a regenerative role in civilisation; he supported monogamy, the single standard, and sexual education. In his view, the "Uranian type" or the "Intermediate type" was innate and inborn, and had a lot to contribute to the evolution of the human race, having a well-developed body and powerful brain. He tried to convey a positive image of homosexuals, presenting them as the balance between the sexes.[87] Finally, Havelock Ellis made a great contribution to sexology in his *Studies in the Psychology of Sex*, seven volumes that appeared between 1897 and 1928. He had previously published in collaboration with J. Addington Symonds *Sexual Inversion* (1897), where they talked about homosexuality as another manifestation of the sexual instinct that could be congenital or acquired both in men and women. They wanted to decriminalise same-sex love and alter public opinion so as to redefine homosexuality in the eyes of the law. Symonds was himself a homosexual and in his short tracts had defined these individuals as those born with an instinctive desire for their own sex.[88]

In this context, Oscar Wilde's prosecution in 1895 under the Labouchère amendment gave publicity to homosexual relations provoking counter-productive results. The affair had political implications and Wilde was sentenced to two years hard labour. The vicious long-term reaction after

---

87 Roy Porter and Lesley Hall, *The Facts of Life: The Creation of Sexual Knowledge in Britain, 1650–1950* (New Haven and London: Yale University Press, 1995), 155–160.
88 Dalley Crozier, "The Medical Construction of Homosexuality and its Relation to the Law in Nineteenth-Century England", 78–80.

the Wilde trial meant that after the trial of the Legitimation League's sole full-time activist, George Bedborough, the so far sole published volume of Ellis's *Studies in the Psychology of Sex* was labelled as "obscene". Ellis responded by publishing this volume and all further volumes in Paris. Life was very tight for sexual deviants from around 1900, and "purity" activists were often part of that narrowing. Even the very careful Carpenter was watched and beset by one or more homophobes. There was fear that imitation of the crime would take place and aspects about it would be openly discussed, spreading its influence to female homosexuality. After Wilde's fall, a section of the Vagrancy Law Amendment Act of 1898 made homosexual solicitation illegal, making "the birch" – flogging – the right punishment for men who became involved in that kind of "love that dare not speak its name".[89] No allusion to either male or female homosexuality is found in the London Lock archives.

According once more to Michel Foucault, sex and sexuality began to be discussed in Victorian discourses, but these discourses were male dominated and did not include the possibility of women participating in debates about law, medicine or politics.[90] As the nineteenth century progressed, women did talk about sexuality when issues of prostitution, white slavery and child abuse were at stake, especially during the Repeal Campaign against the application of the Contagious Diseases Acts of the 1860s and 1870s, and the campaign for the passing of the Criminal Law Amendment Act of the 1880s. However, the possibility of women talking about their own sexuality and sexual experiences was non-existent, and only with the birth of sexology was the path cleared to them as well as to homosexuals and lesbians to express their views openly. Many associations and clubs proliferated like the Men and Women's Club, the Malthusian League and the Legitimation League. The Men and Women's Club was founded by Karl Pearson in 1885 to think about sex. It was formed by professional

---

89   Richard Davenport-Hines, *Sex, Death and Punishment: Attitudes to Sex and Sexuality in Britain since the Renaissance* (London: Fontana Press, 1991), 133–143.
90   Michel Foucault, *The History of Sexuality: Volume I, An Introduction*, trans. Robert Hurley (London: Penguin, 1990), 17–35.

men and middle-class women, both single and married and economically more or less independent, who shared an interest in feminism. It was not a very transgressive group and the male members did not make women's participation comfortable, identifying them as religious and emotional in contrast with their own more rational qualities. The Malthusian League counted also on women among its members in the 1890s, and saw sex as something natural and healthy for women, promoting contraception to avoid illegitimacy but still locating licit intercourse within monogamy. According to their ideas, early marriages would eradicate prostitution and male promiscuity. Free love was becoming popular in certain circles like the Legitimation League established in 1893, which also had a strong representation of women and had its own journal, *The Adult*. The aim of this association was to improve the legal status of bastards combined with criticism of traditional marriage and sexual matters. Another relevant publication was *Shafts: A Paper for Women and the Working Classes*, where issues such as sex education, problem novels, marriage, social purity, prostitution, rational dress, or female chastity were debated both by men and women. There were probably many groups of progressive and anti-conventional people who had broad discussions about all these questions in a less formal way, and women were increasingly taking part in them.[91] Given their informality, they were and are sparsely recorded.

The new century brought several changes to the London Lock, but its spirit remained mostly unchanged. As Pamela Cox argues, the twentieth-century was a continuation of the nineteenth in many aspects concerning the control of venereal disease. This control was exerted by various voluntary, military and statutory powers and through different locations like courts, traditional hospitals, new VD clinics, rescue homes, maternal and infant health centres, military hospitals, etc. Various measures were focused on groups such as pregnant women, mothers, babies, children, soldiers, sailors, delinquent girls and the mentally defective. These groups had in common that they were all subjected to external authority. The methods used for imposing treatment could range from coercive to persuasive.

---

91 Hall, *Sex, Gender, and Social Change in Britain since 1880*, 37, 45, 50–53.

Action continued to be based on voluntarism, with the exception of the two world wars when a system of regulation was put in place, similar to that of the Contagious Diseases Acts. However, the use of salvarsan from the 1910s allowed separating physical cure from moral treatment for the first time in the history of medicine.[92] The London Lock participated in all these shifts, but remained a kind of micro-universe of venereally diseased bodies in the British system till its closure in 1952, supporting the different ideologies behind successive policies. The closure was decided by the North-West Metropolitan Regional Hospital Board on the grounds of "prevention of wasteful overlapping of hospital services",[93] and put an end to a long history of lending service to the outcast, deviant and impure suffering from venereal complaints.

To bring this volume to a close, I would like to emphasise that many of the issues that have been discussed in it have an overwhelming value for the present. Contemporary concerns like prostitution, human trafficking for the purposes of sexual exploitation or child abuse are still painfully present in our contemporary societies, with governments, NGOs and other kinds of agencies being unable to manage the problem on a global, transnational scale. In my view, some of the nineteenth century arguments for the defence of the prostitute as an individual with agency, like those put forward by Josephine Butler, are extremely relevant for the present. Talking about prostitution, she considered it an evil because it caused the destruction of human dignity. Butler was against the idea of its existence as inevitable because this attempted against the rights of women and of the poor. Despite the fact that the prostitute was female, working-class and morally deviant, Butler still believed that she had the right not to be harassed and to choose her own destiny, talking then about female autonomy and resistance to power. Inveighing against the working classes with middle-class norms of domesticity and morality and subjecting them to

---

92 Pamela Cox, "Compulsion, Voluntarism, and Venereal Disease: Governing Sexual Health in England after the Contagious Diseases Acts", *Journal of British Studies* 46, 1 (2007): 92–95.
93 "Closure of the Lock Hospital", *The Lancet*, June 25, 1949: 1109.

different forms of surveillance was probably not the most judicious way to do philanthropy and to contain venereal disease, but at least it meant some steps along the road towards ending the suffering and the horror in the lives of many human beings, in contrast with the too frequent apathy and passivity of our contemporary world.

Nonetheless, the London Lock contributed to the configuration of sexual otherness throughout its history, and can be defined as a space of regulation trying to impose order within the London map of urban sexuality in the Victorian era. As a voluntary institution devoted to the cure of venereal disease and the reform of the deviant female, it reproduced the different forms of social policy that were pervasive during the nineteenth century. It endorsed the various moral and environmental initiatives aimed at controlling the spread of social disorder and disease that were associated with the sexual practices of the depraved and the undeserving poor. In this sense, it is fundamental to acknowledge the role of the London Lock Hospital and Asylum in the construction of sexuality in terms of male and female differences leading to power relations in the fields of social medicine and moral politics, bearing in mind that sexuality is a historically specific and culturally variable notion. And yet, the London Lock was not only the arena where official discourses around sexuality and morality were produced, but also the site, together with a whole range of institutions, of political struggle through the agency exerted by the working class and female and feminist appropriation of particular moral values. Reading between the lines in the archives we can feel the presence of female patients and penitents showing resistance to male authority and middle-class norms.

Bibliography

Archival sources

An Abstract of the Rules and Orders for the Government of the Lock Hospital near Hyde-Park Corner, Instituted July 4, 1746, for the Relief of Venereal Patients Only, By Order of the Annual General Court held April 21, 1814. The Library, Royal College of Surgeons of England, London, MS/0022/5/3.

An Account of the Lock Hospital and Asylum, 1834. The Library, Royal College of Surgeons of England, London, MS0022/3/8.

An Account of the Lock Hospital; to Which is Added an Account of the Lock Asylum, 1835. The Library, Royal College of Surgeons of England, London, MS0022/3/8.

An Account of the Lock Hospital; to Which is Added an Account of the Lock Asylum, 1837. The Library, Royal College of Surgeons of England, London, MS0022/3/8.

An Account of the Nature and Intention of the Lock Asylum, for the Reception of Female Penitents when discharged from the Lock Hospital: with an Abstract of the Accounts, from the first Institution, to LADY-DAY, 1833. Also the Code of the Regulations, with a List of Benefactors and Subscribers. The Library, Royal College of Surgeons of England, London, MS0022/3/8.

Criminal Law Amendment Act, 1885 (An Abstract). The Women's Library, London Metropolitan University, 3/AMS/B/01/01-04, Box 36.

Cuttings Album. The Library, Royal College of Surgeons of England, London, MS0022/11.

Extract from the Annual Report, 1st January, 1855, Cuttings Album. The Library, Royal College of Surgeons of England, London, MS0022/11.

Extract from the Annual Report of the Lock Hospital and Asylum, 1st January, 1860, Cuttings Album. The Library, Royal College of Surgeons of England, London, MS0022/11.

Fifth Annual Report by the Directors of the Glasgow Magdalene Institution, 28 December 1864. Special Collections Department, Glasgow University Library. Accessed December 12, 2009. <http://special.lib.gla.ac.uk/exhibns/month/nov2000.html>.

Hospital House Committee, 1862–1872. The Library, Royal College of Surgeons of England, London, MS0022/2/4/2.

Laws of the London Lock Hospital and Asylum (Rescue Home) 1890. The Library, Royal College of Surgeons of England, London, MS0022/5/11.

Laws of the London Lock Hospital and Asylum, Revised (1840), 1848. The Library, Royal College of Surgeons of England, London, MS0022/5/2.

Lock Asylum Committee (1836–1842). The Library, Royal College of Surgeons of England, London, MS0022/2/1/4.

London Lock Hospital and Asylum Report 1886. The Library, Royal College of Surgeons of England, London, MS0022/4/2.

London Lock Hospital and Asylum Report 1888. The Library, Royal College of Surgeons of England, London, MS0022/4/2.

London Lock Hospital and Asylum Report 1891. The Library, Royal College of Surgeons of England, London, MS0022/4/2.

No 1, Annual Reports in an Octavo Bound Volume, 1789–1828. The Library, Royal College of Surgeons of England, London, MS0022/4/2.

No. 8 Annual Reports in an Octavo Bound Volume, 1873–1893. The Library, Royal College of Surgeons of England, London, MS0022/4/2.

Patients Records, Correspondence and Plates, An Account of the Lock Hospital, from notes taken from the Minute Books. The Library, Royal College of Surgeons of England, London, MS0022/6/3.

Report of the Charities and Religious Societies Connected with the Lock Hospital Chapel 1864. The Library, Royal College of Surgeons of England, London, MS0022/4/1/3.

Report of the Charities and Religious Societies Connected with the Lock Hospital Chapel 1874. The Library, Royal College of Surgeons of England, London, MS0022/4/1/3.

Report of the Charities and Religious Societies Connected with the Lock Hospital Chapel 1876. The Library, Royal College of Surgeons of England, London, MS0022/4/1/3.

Report of the Charities and Religious Societies Connected with the Lock Hospital Chapel 1877. The Library, Royal College of Surgeons of England, London, MS0022/4/1/3.

Report of the Lock Hospital and Asylum for the Years 1868, 1869, 1870, 1871. The Library, Royal College of Surgeons of England, London, MS0022/4/2.

Report of the Lock Hospital, Asylum, and Chapel, 1853. The Library, Royal College of Surgeons of England, London, MS0022/4/2.

Reports of the Lock Hospital, Asylum, and Chapel, 1856, 1857, 1858, 1859, 1860. The Library, Royal College of Surgeons of England, London, MS0022/4/2.

Rules for Patients in Hospital. The Library, Royal College of Surgeons of England, London, MS0022/5/3.

Stead, W.T. "The Maiden Tribute of Modern Babylon", *Pall Mall Gazette*, July 6, 1885. The Women's Library, London Metropolitan University, 3/AMS/B/01/01-04, Box 36.

Stead, W.T. "The Maiden Tribute of Modern Babylon", *Pall Mall Gazette*, July 10, 1885. The Women's Library, London Metropolitan University, 3/AMS/B/01/01-04, Box 36.

Primary and secondary sources

Acton, William. 1857a. *The Functions and Disorders of the Reproductive Organs, in Childhood, Youth, Adult Age, and Advanced Life, Considered in the Physiological, Social, and Moral Relations*. London: John Churchill, New Burlington Street.

——. 1857b. *Prostitution Considered in its Moral, Social and Sanitary Aspects, in London and other Large Cities with Proposals for the Mitigation and Prevention of its Attendant Evils*, London: John Churchill, New Burlington Street.

Andrew, Donna. 1991. "Two Medical Charities in Nineteenth-Century London: The Lock Hospital and the Lying-In Charity for Married Women". In *Medicine and Charity before the Welfare State*, edited by Jonathan Barry and Colin Jones, 82–97. London: Routledge.

Atwood, Nina. 2011. *The Prostitute's Body: Rewriting Prostitution in Victorian Britain*. London: Pickering and Chatto.

Bartley, Paula. 1998. "Preventing Prostitution: The Ladies' Association for the Care and Protection of Young Girls in Birmingham, 1887–1914". *Women's History Review*, 7 (1): 37–60.

——. 2000. *Prostitution: Prevention and Reform in England, 1860–1914*. London and New York: Routledge.

Beckett Truman, Edgar, MD. "The Contagious Diseases Acts. To the Editor of the Lancet". *The Lancet*, 18 November 1882: 871.

Bell, Benjamin. 1793. *Treatise on Gonorrhoea and Lues Venerea*. London: John Murray, Fleet Street.

Bland, Lucy. 1992. "'Purifying' the Public World: Feminist Vigilantes in Late Victorian England". *Women History Review*, 1 (3): 397–412.

——. 2002. *Banishing the Beast: Feminism, Sex and Morality*. London and New York: Tauris Parke Paperbacks.

Bourdieu, Pierre. 1977. *Outline of a Theory Practice*. Translated by R. Nice. Cambridge: Cambridge University Press.

Boyd, Nancy. 1982. *Josephine Butler, Octavia Hill, Florence Nightingale: Three Victorian Women who Changed the World*. London: The Macmillan Press.

Bruce, Alexander. 1868. *An Epitome of the Venereal Diseases being a Succinct Account of the Well Established and More Important Facts to these Diseases*. London: H.K. Lewis, of Gower Street.

Butler, A.S.G. 1954. *Portrait of Josephine Butler*. London: Faber and Faber.

Butler, J.E. 1910. *Personal Reminiscences of a Great Crusade*. London: Horace Marshall and Son.

"Chancroid". Accessed March 8, 2009 at <http://www.idph.state.il.us/public/hb/hbchancroid.htm>.

Cherry, Steven. 2000. "Hospital Sunday, Workplace Collections, and Issues in Late Nineteenth-Century Hospital Funding". *Medical History*, 44: 461–488.

"Closure of the Lock Hospital". *The Lancet*, June 25, 1949: 1109.

Cox, Pamela. 2007. "Compulsion, Voluntarism, and Venereal Disease: Governing Sexual Health in England after the Contagious Diseases Acts". *Journal of British Studies*, 46 (1): 91–115.

Dalley Crozier, Ivan. 2001. "The Medical Construction of Homosexuality and its Relation to the Law in Nineteenth-Century England". *Medical History*, 45: 61–82.

Davenport-Hines, Richard. 1991. *Sex, Death and Punishment: Attitudes to Sex and Sexuality in Britain since the Renaissance*. London: Fontana Press.

Davidoff, Leonore, and Catherine Hall. 1992. *Family Fortunes: Men and Women of the English Middle Class 1780–1850*. London: Routledge.

D'Cruze, Shani. 1998. *Crimes of Outrage: Sex, Violence and Victorian Working Women*. London: UCL Press.

Dillon, Patrick. 2003. "The Roots of Reform". *History Today*, 57 (3): 44–46.

"Extension of the Contagious Diseases Act of 1866 to the Civil Population". *The Lancet*, July 4, 1868: 21–22.

Fessler, A. 1946. "Leaflets on the Treatment of Venereal Diseases of the Early Nineteenth Century". *British Journal of Venereal Disease* 22 (2): 85–89.

———. 1949. "Advertisements on the Treatment of Venereal Disease and the Social History of Venereal Disease". *British Journal of Venereal Disease*, 25 (2): 84–87.

———. 1951. "Venereal Disease and Prostitution in the Reports of the Poor Law Commissioners, 1834–1850". *British Journal of Venereal Disease*, 27 (3): 154–157.

Fessler, A., and R. Sharpe. 1947. "Advertisements on the Treatment of Venereal Diseases in the Eighteenth and Nineteenth Centuries". *British Journal of Venereal Disease*, 23 (3): 125–127.

Finnegan, Frances. 1979. *Poverty and Prostitution: A Study of Victorian Prostitutes in York*. Cambridge: Cambridge University Press.

———. 1991. *Do Penance or Perish: A Study of Magdalene Asylums in Ireland*. Piltown, Co. Kilkenny: Congrave Press.

Foucault, Michel. 1979. *Discipline and Punish: The Birth of a Prison*. Translated by Alan Sheridan. London: Penguin Books.

———. 1990. *The History of Sexuality: Volume I, An Introduction*. Translated by Robert Hurley. London: Penguin.

"Genital Warts". Accessed March 3, 2009. <http://kidshealth.org/parent/inefections/std/genital_warts.html#cat20046>.

"Gonorrhoea: Symptoms and Treatments". Accessed March 3, 2009. <http://www.ivillage.co.uk/print/0,9688,665001,00.html>.

Gorham, Deborah. 1978. "The 'Maiden Tribute of Modern Babylon' Re-examined: Child Prostitution and the Idea of Childhood in Late-Victorian England". *Victorian Studies*, 21 (3): 353–379.

Hall, Lesley. 2004. "Hauling Down the Double Standard: Feminism, Social Purity and Sexual Science in Late Nineteenth Century Britain". *Gender and History*, 16 (1): 36–56.

———. 2013. *Sex, Gender, and Social Change in Britain since 1880*. 2nd ed. London: Palgrave Macmillan.

Harrison, Fraser. 1977. *The Dark Angel: Aspects of Victorian Sexuality*. London: Sheldon Press.

Harrison, L.W. 1931. *The Diagnosis and Treatment of Venereal Diseases in General Practice*. 2nd ed. Oxford: Oxford University Press.

Higgs, Michelle. 2009. *Life in the Victorian Hospital*. Stroud, Gloucestershire: The History Press.

Howell, Philip. 2000. "A Private Contagious Diseases Act: Prostitution and Public Space in Victorian Cambridge". *Journal of Historical Geography*, 26 (3): 376–402.

———. 2009. *Geographies of Regulation: Policing Prostitution in Nineteenth-Century Britain and the Empire*. Cambridge: Cambridge University Press.

Hunter, John. 1786. *On the Venereal Disease*. London: Castle Street, Leicester Square.

Innes Williams, David. 1995. *The London Lock: A Charitable Hospital for Venereal Disease, 1746–1952*. London and New York: Royal Society of Medicine Press Ltd.

Irwin, Mary Ann. 1998. "White Slavery As Metaphor Anatomy of Moral Panic". Accessed August 23, 2013. <http://userwww.sfsu.edu/epf/journal_archive/volume_V,_1996/irwin_m.pdf>.

Jackson, Louise. 2000. *Child Sexual Abuse in Victorian England*. London and New York: Routledge.

Jones, Steve. 1994. *London … The Sinister Side*. Nottingham: Wicked Publications.

Kidd, Alan. 1999. *State, Society and the Poor in Nineteenth-Century England*. London: Macmillan Press.

Laite, J. 2006. *Paying the Price again: Prostitution Policy in Historical Perspective*. Accessed May 5, 2008. <http://www.historyandpolicy.org/papers/policy-paper-46.html>.

Lane, James R., F.R.C.S. "Remarks on the Cases Admitted into the London Female Lock Hospital during the Year 1867". *The British Medical Journal*, 1 (372), February 15, 1868: 139–140.

———. "Notes on the Practice of the London Female Lock Hospital". *The British Medical Journal*, 2 (414), December 5, 1868: 592.

Lees, Robert. 1961. "The 'Lock Wards' of Edinburgh Royal Infirmary". *British Journal of Venereal Disease*, 37 (3): 187–189.

Leitch, Vincent B., ed. 2001. *The Norton Anthology of Theory and Criticism*. New York and London: W-W-W Norton and Company.

Levine, Philippa. 2003. *Prostitution, Race and Politics: Policing Venereal Disease in the British Empire*. London and New York: Routledge.

Lignum, John. 1819. *Treatise on Venereal and Syphilitic Diseases; Containing Plain and Practical Directions for the Effectual Cure of all Degrees of the above Complaints; with Observations on the Uses and Abuses of Mercury Intended for the Instruction of General Readers*. Manchester: T. Rogerson.

Logan, William. 1871. *The Great Social Evil; its Causes, Extent, Results and Remedies*. London: Hodder and Stoughton.

Lond, M.D., D.P.H. Cantab. "Treatment in Infirmary Lock Wards". *The British Medical Journal*, November 24, 1900: 1537.

"London City Mission". Accessed August 22, 2013. <http://www.lcm.org.uk/Groups/8868/London_City_Mission/About_Us/History/History.aspx.>

Longmate, Norman. 2003. *The Workhouse: A Social History*. London: Pimlico.

Lowndes, Frederick W., M.R.C.S. Eng. "The Liverpool Lock Hospital and the Prevalence and Severity of Constitutional Syphilis in Liverpool". *The British Medical Journal*, 1 (1011), 15 May 1880: 727–729.

———. 1882. *Lock Hospitals and Lock Wards in General Hospitals*, London: J. & A. Churchill; Liverpool: Adam Holden.

———. "Lock Hospitals and Lock Wards. To the Editors of *The Lancet*". *The Lancet*, April 1, 1899: 927.

Mahood, Linda. 1990. *The Magdalenes: Prostitution in the Nineteenth Century*. London and New York: Routledge.

Marshik, Celia. 2006. *British Modernism and Censorship*. Cambridge: Cambridge University Press.

McDonald, Lynn, ed. 2005. *Florence Nightingale on Women, Medicine, Midwifery and Prostitution*. Ontario: Wilfrid Laurier University Press.

Mc Hugh, Paul. 1980. *Prostitution and Victorian Social Reform*. London: Croom Helm.

Mason, Michael. 1995a. *The Making of Victorian Sexual Attitudes*. Oxford and New York: Oxford University Press.
———. 1995b. *The Making of Victorian Sexuality*, Oxford and New York: Oxford University Press.
Mayhew, Henry. 1851. *London Labour and the London Poor*. London: Charles Griffin and Company.
Merions, Linda, ed. 1997. *The Secret Malady: Venereal Disease in Eighteenth Century Britain and France*. Lexington, Kentucky: University of Kentucky Press.
Mitchell, Sally. 1981. *The Fallen Angel: Chastity, Class and Women's Reading 1835–1880*. Bowling Green, Ohio: Bowling Green University Popular Press.
Moberly Bell, E. 1962. *Josephine Butler: Flame of Fire*. London: Constable and Co. Ltd.
Mort, Frank. 2000. *Dangerous Sexualities: Medico-Moral Politics in England since 1830*. 2nd ed. Routledge: London and New York.
Mumm, Susan. 1996. "'Not Worse than Other Girls': The Convent-based Rehabilitation of Fallen Women in Victorian Britain". *Journal of Social History*, 29 (3): 527–546.
Nead, Lynda. 1988. *Myths of Sexuality: Representations of Women in Victorian Britain*. London: Blackwell.
———. 1999. "From Alleys to Courts: Obscenity and the Mapping of Mid-Victorian London". *New Formations: A Journal of Culture/Theory/Politics: Sexual Geographies*, 37: 33–46.
Oswald, Janet. 2012. "The Spinning House Girls: Cambridge University's Distinctive Policing of Prostitution, 1823–1894". *Urban History*, 39 (3): 453–470.
Parent-Duchatelet, A.J.B. 1836. *De la Prostitution dans la Ville de Paris*. Paris: J.B. Bailliere et Fils.
Payne, Jennifer. "The Criminal Law Amendment Act of 1885 and Sexual Assault on Minors". Accessed September 13, 2009. <http://www.geocities.com/Athens/Aegean/7023/Consent.html>.
Pearson, John. 1800. *Observations on Various Items of Materia Medica Used in the Treatment of Lues Venerea*. London: W. Smith.
Peers, Douglas M., 1998. "Soldiers, Surgeons and the Campaign to Combat Sexually Transmitted Disease in Colonial India, 1805–1860". *Medical History*, 42 (2): 137–160.
Perkin, Joan. 1994. *Victorian Women*. Cambridge: Cambridge University Press.
Pharmacopeia in Use at the Male and Out-Patient Department of the London Lock Hospital. 1887. London: Adlard and Son, Bartholomew Close.
Poovey, Mary. 1989. *Uneven Developments: The Ideological Work of Gender in Mid-Victorian England*. London: Virago Press.

Porter, Roy, and Lesley Hall. 1995. *The Facts of Life: The Creation of Sexual Knowledge in Britain, 1650–1950*. New Haven and London: Yale University Press.

Purvis, J. 1991. *A History of Women's Education in England*. Buckingham: Open University Press.

———, ed. 1998. *Women's History: Britain, 1850–1945: An Introduction*. London and New York: Routledge.

"Reminiscences of the Liverpool Lock Hospital". *The Lancet*, February 2, 1907: 305–306.

"Report on the Northleach Workhouse and Infirmary". *The British Medical Journal*, November 16, 1867: 458–459.

"Report on the Workhouse Infirmary of Clifton". *The British Medical Journal*, November 9, 1867: 433.

Ricord, Philippe. 1938. *Traité Practique sur les Maladies Vénériennes*. Paris: Librairie des Sciences Medicales, De Just Rouvier et E.Le Bouvier.

Rimke, Heidi. 2003. "Constituting Transgressive Interiorities: Nineteenth Century Readings of Morally Mad Bodies". In *Violence and the Body: Race, Gender and the State*, edited by Arturi J. Aldama, 247–262. Bloomington, IN, USA: Indiana University Press.

Romero Ruiz, Maria Isabel. 2011. "Women's Identity and Migration: Stead's Articles in the *Pall Mall Gazette* on Prostitution and White Slavery". In *Cultural Migrations and Gendered Subjects: Colonial and Postcolonial Representations of the Female Body*, edited by Silvia P. Castro Borrego and Maria Isabel Romero Ruiz, 27–53. Newcastle-upon-Tyne: Cambridge Scholars Publishing.

Ross, S.J. "The Liverpool Lock Hospital. To the Editors of *The Lancet*". *The Lancet*, April 22, 1899: 1120.

Savage, Gail. 1990. "'The Wilful Communication of a Loathsome Disease': Marital Conflict and Venereal Disease in Victorian England". *Victorian Studies*, 34 (1): 35–54.

A Short History of the London Lock Hospital and Rescue Home, 1746–1906. The Library, Royal College of Surgeons of England, London.

Siena, Kevin. 2004. *Venereal Disease Hospitals and the Urban Poor: London's Foul Wards 1600–1800*. Rochester: University of Rochester Press.

Sigsworth, E.M. and Wyke, T.J. 1973. "A Study of Victorian Prostitution and Venereal Disease". In *Suffer and Be Still: Women in the Victorian Age*, edited by Martha Vicinus, 77–99. Bloomington & London: Indiana University Press.

Smith, F.B. 1990. "The Contagious Diseases Acts Reconsidered". *The Society for the Social History of Medicine*, 3: 197–215.

Smith, James M. 2008. *Ireland's Magdalene Laundries and the Nation's Architecture of Containment*. Manchester: Manchester University Press.

Spongberg, Mary. 1997. *Feminising Venereal Disease: The Body of the Prostitute in Nineteenth Century Medical Discourse*. London: Macmillan.
Stevenson, Kim. "Observations on the Law Relating to Sexual Offences: the Historic Scandal of Women's Silences". Accessed July 27, 2010. <http://webjcli.ncl.ac.uk/1999/issue4/stevenson4.html>.
"Syphilis". Accessed August 8, 2012. <http://kidshealth.org/parent/infections/std/syphilis.html#cat20046>.
Tait, William. 1841 *Magdalenism: An Enqiry into the Extent, Causes, and Consequences of Prostitution in Edinburgh*. Edinburgh: P. Rickard, South Bridge.
Temperley, Nicholas. 1993. "The Lock Hospital Chapel and its Music". *Journal of the Royal Music Association*, 118 (1): 44–72.
Walkowitz, Judith R. 1982. "Male Vice and Female Virtue: Feminism and the Politics of Prostitution in Nineteenth-Century Britain". *History Workshop Journal*, 13: 79–93.
———. 1991. *Prostitution and Victorian Society: Women, Class and the State*. Cambridge: Cambridge University Press.
———. 1992. *City of Dreadful Delight: Narratives of Sexual Danger in Late-Victorian London*. London: Virago Press.
Weisz, George. 2003. "The Emergence of Medical Specialization in the Nineteenth Century". *Bulletin of the History of Medicine*, 77 (3): 536–764.
Wilson Carpenter, Mary. 2010. *Health, Medicine and Society in Victorian England*. Oxford: ABC Clio.
Wyke, T.J. 1973. "Hospital Facilities for, and Diagnosis and Treatment of, Venereal Disease in England, 1800–1870". *British Journal of Venereal Disease*, 49 (1): 78–85.
———. 1975. "The Manchester and Salford Lock Hospital, 1818–1917". *Medical History*, 19 (1): 73–86.
Young, Arlene. 2008. "'Entirely a Woman's Question?': Class, Gender, and the Victorian Nurse". *Journal of Victorian Culture*, 13 (1): 18–41.

Index

abolition 119, 120, 123
abolitionists 120, 121, 179
abortion 33
abuse 174, 184
Act to Protect Women under Twenty-one from Fraudulent Practices for Procuring their Defilement (1849) 175
Acton, William 31, 32, 33, 44, 97, 109
Addington Symonds, John 195
Admiralty 103, 104, 105, 106, 107, 149
adultery 28, 46, 76
age of consent 35, 54, 89, 121, 175, 176, 177, 182
agency 8, 71, 114, 198, 199
angel in the house 171
annual subscriptions 7
apothecaries 4, 13, 16, 51, 60, 66
archives 1, 2, 64, 69, 98, 99, 100, 132, 133, 196, 199
asexual 25, 119
Association for Promoting the Extension of the Contagious Diseases Acts (the Extensionist Association) 109, 110
asylums 2, 3, 8, 11, 22, 23, 24, 29, 53, 54, 55, 58, 59, 62, 63, 64, 65, 67, 70, 76, 78, 84, 86, 87, 92, 98, 99, 100, 108, 114, 120, 125, 126, 127, 129, 130, 131, 132, 133, 134, 135, 136, 137, 139, 140, 141, 142, 143, 144, 145, 146, 147, 148, 149, 150, 151, 152, 153, 154, 155, 157, 160, 161, 162, 171, 187, 188, 189, 191, 199

Band of Hope Mission, the 164
bastard 14, 197; bastardy 121
behavior 9, 25, 26, 58, 63, 64, 68, 70, 71, 74, 79, 80, 81, 89, 97, 98, 106, 107, 125, 129, 132, 133, 135, 137, 141, 145, 147, 151, 154, 155, 156, 166, 172
benefactions 60
benefactors 7, 59, 62, 99
bequests 7
birth control *see* contraception
bonds 12
Bordo, Susan 39, 114
Bourdieu, Pierre 173
British Hospitals Association 191
British Medical Journal, the 123
Bromfield, William 14, 16, 20, 22, 128
brothels 10, 34, 90, 109, 124, 150, 175, 177, 178, 181, 182, 185, 186
brothel-keepers 34, 90, 104, 122, 177, 178
brothel-owners 178, 182
Bruce, H.A. 122, 177
buggery 194
Butler, Josephine 116, 118, 120, 121, 122, 123, 176, 177, 178, 182, 184, 198

carceral, the 8
Carpenter, Edward 195, 196
chancres 37, 187; syphilitic 40
chancroid 36, 38, 54, 87
chaplains 1, 16, 19, 20, 22, 60, 61, 62, 65, 78, 86, 124, 133, 134, 162, 189; chaplaincy 21
charities 6, 7, 8, 11, 16, 17, 18, 19, 21, 22, 24, 28, 72, 85, 102, 110, 126, 127,

128, 130, 132, 133, 134, 135, 137, 138,
140, 143, 144, 145, 149, 156, 168,
169, 190
charity movement 3
Charity Organisation Society 191
charity work 13
chastity 25, 26, 28, 159, 165, 166, 167, 179,
197
child abuse 171, 172, 173, 174, 177, 183,
185, 196, 198
child prostitution *see under* prostitution
child rape 173
childbirth 37, 187
children's sexuality 186
church collections 7
Church Penitentiary Association 10
Clapham Sect 10, 130
claps 40, 48
classification 9, 30, 144, 160
commodity 27
compassion 10, 17, 18, 28, 29, 146
congregation 20, 21
contagion 16, 17, 18, 28, 34, 37, 39, 40,
43, 44, 45, 57, 75, 93, 96, 113,
119, 129
Contagious Diseases Acts 3, 24, 31, 32,
81, 85, 92, 94, 95, 97, 98, 101, 102,
103, 104, 106, 107, 108, 109, 110,
164, 171, 176, 177, 186, 188,
196, 198
contamination 19, 31, 39, 42, 45, 57, 168
continence 159
contraception 33, 184, 185, 195, 197
contributions 1, 22, 132, 161, 169, 188, 192
contributors 108, 188, 193
corruption 28, 39, 44, 57, 114, 119, 136,
142, 148, 168, 172, 173, 177, 178
Criminal Law Amendment Act
(1885) 35, 124, 151, 182, 185, 186,
193, 196
Custody of Children Act (1891) 183

debauchery 29
decency 3, 14, 19, 23, 30, 32, 44, 46, 57,
58, 62, 72, 74, 75, 81, 107, 109, 114,
129, 135, 136, 151, 186
delicacy 26
delivery 100
dependency 26
depravity 29, 32, 39, 44, 45, 81, 82, 94,
102, 144, 156, 160–161, 167–1688,
172, 177, 199
deserving poor 156
destitute, the 10, 13, 17, 18, 80, 91, 102,
106, 143, 161, 177
destitution 32, 84
deviants 2, 9, 26, 27, 57, 58, 61, 74, 75, 78,
80, 85, 92, 126, 130, 132, 142, 147,
157, 172, 173, 174, 196, 198
discipline 8, 14, 57, 72, 91, 99, 102, 126,
130, 136, 137, 139, 140, 141, 147,
149, 151, 155, 193
discourses 8, 27, 28, 31, 32, 57, 58, 63, 68,
75, 81, 94, 114, 119, 130, 132, 137,
163, 173, 194, 196, 199
discrimination 102, 118, 157
dispensaries 6
districts 24
docile bodies 8, 9, 137, 141
docility 53
domestication 143, 157
domestic environment 128
domestic ideology 25, 186
domesticity 25, 97, 126, 132, 167, 198
donations 7, 11, 16, 60, 124, 127, 128, 130,
143, 152, 154, 188, 191, 192
donors 15, 132, 161, 188
double spheres 25
double standard 23, 25, 58, 119, 122, 164,
173
downward path 21, 28, 31, 32
dreadful distemper 58
drunkenness 27, 57

Index

Elizabethan Poor Law (1601) 12
emigration 32
erotic 83
Evangelical Movement 126
Evangelicalism 82, 126, 130, 163
Evangelicals 10, 15, 22, 130, 136, 164, 171
evil courses 90, 133, 134, 135, 155
examination 96, 103, 107, 111, 114, 117, 122, 123
extension 106, 107, 109, 110, 111

fall 30, 90, 173, 196
fallen, the 134, 136, 184
fallen angels 116
fallen women 1, 2, 3, 23, 26, 55, 58, 61, 81, 116, 121–122, 126, 127, 128, 130, 132, 136, 142, 143, 146, 147, 148, 150, 152, 157, 160, 161, 163, 171; fallen working-class sisters 117
female sexuality 2, 25, 55, 93–94, 119, 166, 173, 174, 194
femininity 25, 26, 143
feminism 116, 118, 119, 120, 148, 159, 164–165, 168, 181, 183, 184, 186, 193–194, 197, 199
fertility 27
flogging 196
Foucauldian 8, 85, 141, 145
Foucault, Michel 9, 27, 30, 114, 136, 196
foul disease 11, 19, 39, 45, 50, 52, 54
foul patients 1, 9, 13, 24, 71
foul wards 7, 13
Friendly Societies 192
funding 2, 7, 11, 14, 17, 57, 59, 124, 127, 149, 160, 186, 188, 190
funds 20, 24, 60, 152, 188, 192, 193

Garrison towns 24, 104, 107, 112, 149
Geddes, Patrick and Arthur Thomson 194, 195

gender 2, 9, 11, 12, 55, 58, 63, 68, 74, 86, 88, 93, 126, 129, 130, 132, 136, 157, 167, 172, 174
General Medical Council 5
genital examination 94, 96
Girls' Friendly Society 164
gonorrhoea 36, 37, 38, 40, 41, 42, 48, 49, 51, 54, 67, 87, 112, 113, 187
Governors 1, 7, 12, 14, 15, 16, 19, 22, 54, 59, 62, 66, 72, 73, 84, 85, 86, 127, 128, 134, 135, 143, 154, 188, 192
Great Social Evil 27, 30, 91, 97, 109, 125
Greg, W.R. 97
Guaiacum 50

Hanway, Jonas 127, 128
Harveian Medical Society 109
Havelock Ellis, Henry 193, 195, 196
hierarchy 30, 66, 93, 119, 141, 145, 151
Hind, Rev. W.H. 86, 87, 89, 90, 91, 148, 149
homophobes 196
homosexuality 93, 106, 182, 193, 194, 195, 196
Hopkins, Ellis 164, 182
Hospital Saturday 192
Hospital Sunday 192
Houses of Mercy 147, 148
human trafficking 198
humours 8, 47
Hunter, John 15, 40, 44

illegitimacy 197
illegitimate children 26, 167
illegitimate mothers 101
immoral 14, 82, 85, 107, 128, 129, 150, 160, 177, 183, 184
immorality 28, 57, 74, 81, 106, 110, 114, 117, 119, 121, 129, 155, 161, 165, 173, 175, 184
impure 97, 198

impure intercourse 40, 44
incest 82, 147, 174, 175, 183, 184
indecency 182
indoctrination 23, 61, 127, 135, 136
Industrial Schools 111, 177, 183
Industrial Schools Act (1866) 177
Industrial Schools Act (1868) 144
Industrial Schools Act (1880) 177, 183
industriousness 128, 136
infanticide 3
infection 13, 37, 38, 40, 41, 44, 45, 53, 57, 93, 106, 110, 191
infertility 33 *see also* sterility
infirmaries 6, 11, 102, 122, 190
inmates 8, 11, 12, 13, 21, 23, 53, 57, 63, 68, 71, 72, 74, 79, 87, 88, 89, 91, 92, 100, 102, 125, 128, 131, 133, 136, 137, 140, 141, 142, 143, 144, 145, 146, 147, 149, 151, 152, 153, 157, 160, 162, 171, 188
innocence 172, 173, 174, 175, 181
innocent 16, 18, 46, 85, 96, 102, 161, 168, 171, 172, 180
inspection 93, 103, 112, 113, 114, 118, 135, 149, 150, 161, 186
instructions 23, 60, 61, 71, 72, 78, 79, 91, 92, 99, 107, 108, 133, 135, 141, 149, 152, 155, 162, 164, 166, 169
insubordination 9
intemperance 29, 90, 156
intercourse 40, 47, 118, 173, 176, 197
International Bureau for the Suppression of the Traffic in Persons (1899) 182
isolation 126, 135, 136, 154, 156
itch ward 102

juvenile prostitution *see under* prostitution

Kinnaird, Arthur 162, 163, 191
knowledge 8, 81, 82, 114, 136, 137

Labouchère amendment 194, 195
lack of morals 40, 89, 164
Ladies' Association for the Care of Friendless Girls 164, 165, 170
Ladies' Committee 63, 65, 125, 134, 137, 162, 189
Ladies' Manifesto *see* Women's Protest
Ladies' National Association for the Repeal of the Contagious Diseases Acts 115, 116, 120, 122, 123, 184–185
lady subscribers 16
Lancet, The 123
Lane, Dr. James 112, 113, 114
laundresses 148
laundry 65, 140
laundry-work 73, 131, 140, 141, 144, 147, 151,
legacies 16, 143, 151, 191
Legitimation League 196, 197
lepers 39
lesbianism 141, 194, 196
licentiousness 17, 29, 43
Local Government Act (1871) 159
lock 11, 15, 16, 17, 18, 19, 20, 21, 23, 24, 25, 28, 29, 32, 39, 41, 43, 48, 51, 52, 53, 58, 59, 60, 62, 63, 64, 64, 65, 66, 67, 69, 70, 71, 72, 73, 74, 75, 76, 79, 80, 81, 83, 84, 85, 86, 87, 92, 96, 97, 100, 102, 103, 106, 108, 110, 111, 112, 115, 120, 121, 124, 125, 126, 127, 128, 129, 130, 132, 133, 134, 135, 136, 137, 139, 141, 142, 143, 145, 148, 149, 150, 151, 152, 153, 154, 155, 159, 160, 161, 163, 167, 168, 169, 171, 175, 186, 187, 188, 189, 190, 191, 193, 197, 198, 199
lock accommodation 109
lock facilities 107, 109
lock wards 2, 24, 48–49, 102, 190
Logan, William 30, 91
loitering 35

Index

London Committee for the Suppression of the Traffic in British Girls for the Purposes of Continental Prostitution 178
London Society for the Protection of Females and the Prevention of Juvenile Prostitution 175
low orders 10, 75, 102, 129, 142, 150, 156, 171, 180

Madan, Martin 19, 20, 21, 22
Magdalene 127, 128, 129, 130, 132, 143, 144, 145, 146, 148, 150, 151, 161, 165, 166
Magdalene laundry 157
male continence 97
male desire 119, 120
male lust 120
male sexual impulses 118
male sexuality 164, 184
Malthusian League 196, 197
Martineau, Harriet 96, 116
masculinity 74
masturbation 82, 83, 168, 184
Matrimonial Causes Act (1857) 46
matron 13, 60, 62, 63, 64, 65, 68, 69, 70, 74, 79, 86, 98, 99, 125, 131, 133, 135, 137, 141, 142, 145, 149, 151, 152, 153, 154, 155, 156, 157, 162, 188
Mayhew, Henry 30
Medical Act (1858) 4
medical authorities 15, 41, 42, 50, 55, 65, 93, 97, 107, 115
medical examination 93, 103, 111, 118
medical inspection 94, 96, 103
medical officers 65, 66, 70, 74, 189
medical press 6
medical profession 4, 20, 44, 45, 82, 92, 123
medical reform 7
Medical Register 5, 128

medical schools 4, 5, 190
medical staff 71, 72, 85, 108, 125, 191
medical students 5, 8, 12, 66, 86, 187, 190
Men and Women's Club 196
menstruation 40
mercury 47, 49, 50, 51, 52, 53, 54, 87, 187; mercurial methods 48; mercurial treatment 50
Methodism 21
Metropolitan Police Act (1839) 35
miasma 44, 45
misbehavior 76, 156
miscarriages 27
misconduct 99
missionaries 108, 162
missionary work 163
moral 25, 31, 32, 46, 48, 49, 57, 58, 75, 76, 82, 84, 90, 93, 108, 109, 111, 114, 115, 119, 124, 126, 128, 129, 130, 132, 140, 143, 144, 149, 150, 155, 163, 165, 172, 174, 178, 199
moral character 68
moral contagion 12, 140
moral corruption 39, 102, 134, 142
moral cure 22
morality 10, 12, 28, 58, 69, 81, 82, 83, 86, 89, 92, 97, 106, 123, 130, 144, 156, 157, 164, 165, 198, 199
moral panic 181
moral reform 12, 22, 126, 163
moral reformation 61, 128 ; moral reformers 15, 89
moral sinners 15
moral transgression 14
moral values 26, 28, 74, 164, 199

National Association for the Repeal of the Contagious Diseases Acts 115, 116
National Health Service 193

National Medical Association for the Repeal of the Contagious Diseases Acts 122
National Vigilance Association (1885) 182, 183, 184, 185, 186
needle-women 142, 149
needle-work 73, 79, 131, 139, 141, 166
Nevins, Dr. John 122, 123
New Poor Law (1834) 101
Nightingale, Florence 69, 96, 116, 117, 118
non-contaminant 23
nurses 13, 15, 18, 60, 62, 63, 65, 68, 69, 70, 71, 73, 75, 79, 102, 189, 190, 191

Obscene Publications Act (1857) 83
obscenity 83, 185, 186, 196
Offences against the Person Act (1861) 176, 177
other, the 74, 107, 130
outcast 28, 145, 172
outhouses 7, 11, 15
Out-patient Department 24, 67, 84, 85, 191
over-crowding 28, 82
Oxford Movement, the 10

Pall Mall Gazette 182
parasyphilitic disease 36
parishes 12, 13, 14, 17, 53, 72, 87, 100, 101, 105, 124, 144, 145, 155
parish relief 12
passing 13
patriarchal 28, 74, 119, 120
patronage 5
Pearson, Karl 196
Pearson, John 51, 53
Pelvic Inflammatory Disease 37, 42
penitential system 10
penitentiaries 2, 8, 10, 74, 101, 127, 132, 146, 147, 148, 152, 157, 161

penitents 3, 22, 78, 84, 86, 125, 130, 131, 133, 135, 136, 137, 141, 143, 145, 146, 147, 148, 149, 150, 151, 153, 155, 160, 199
periodical examination 107, 121
perverts 194
philanthropists 6, 10, 22, 33, 163, 193
philanthropy 6, 28, 55, 58, 80, 116, 143, 164, 188, 189, 199
physical contagion 12
physical cure 22
physicians 4, 8, 13, 16, 51, 54, 60, 65, 66, 67, 73, 86, 187
pimps 35, 36
police 93, 106
policing 2, 24, 44
policy 81, 92, 126, 132, 155, 159, 183, 184, 192, 198, 199
pollution 106, 114, 121, 124; pollutants 44, 82
Poor Law 5
Poor Law Infirmaries 1, 12
poor relief 12
pornography 83, 184, 185
power 8, 9, 10, 71, 81, 83, 105, 109, 111, 119, 129, 132, 136, 137, 141, 155, 157, 164, 171, 173, 181, 197, 198, 199
pox, the 1, 13, 17, 39
pregnancy 13, 27, 99, 101, 111, 134, 142, 151, 166, 197
premarital sex 13, 25, 26
Prince of Wales Hospital Fund 193
private sphere 63, 74, 144
probation 135, 149; probationers 69, 189
Proclamation Society 10
procurement 35; procurers 177, 180
profligacy 18, 22
promiscuity 17, 45, 74–75, 94, 127, 129, 144, 166, 172, 185197
propriety 75

Index

prostitutes 2, 3, 9, 10, 16, 17, 18, 23, 26, 28, 29, 30, 31, 32, 33, 34, 35, 36, 43, 44, 45, 46, 47, 53, 58, 61, 82, 88, 89, 90, 93, 93, 94, 95, 96, 97, 101, 102, 103, 104, 107, 108, 110, 111, 114, 118, 119, 120, 121, 122, 124, 127, 128, 129, 130, 132, 144, 147, 148, 150, 151, 160, 161, 163, 173, 175, 177, 178, 179, 180, 184, 185, 186, 198; common prostitutes 27, 35, 103, 107; streetwalkers 34, 95, 101
prostitution 10, 21, 27, 28, 29, 30, 31, 32, 33, 35, 45, 48, 55, 61, 81, 88, 89, 91, 92, 93, 94, 95, 97, 107, 109, 110, 116, 117, 118, 120, 121, 122, 126, 143, 147, 149, 150, 164, 165, 166, 167, 172, 174, 175, 176, 179, 180, 182, 184, 185, 197, 198; child prostitution 3, 172, 173, 175, 176, 177, 179; juvenile prostitution 172, 179, 182
Protection of Children's Act (1889) 183
prudery 174
Public Health Act (1848) 81
public space 148
public sphere 11, 25, 28, 141, 189
punishment 9, 61, 71, 72, 93, 102, 103, 107, 115, 119, 121, 128, 136, 137, 147, 155, 156
Punishment of Incest Act (1908) 183
purify 148, 164, 186
puritanism 10
purity 3, 23, 26, 97, 119, 124, 132, 163, 164, 165–166, 168, 178, 182, 185, 186, 194, 196, 197

quacks 3, 5, 48, 83

rape 29, 89, 147, 172, 173, 174, 180; of the speculum, the 118
rates 12
rebellion 132, 154

rebelliousness 156
redemption 61, 126, 127, 130, 145
reform 2, 10, 23, 55, 76, 80, 97, 110, 121, 126, 127, 128, 143, 147, 148, 157, 159, 161, 162, 164, 167, 177, 179, 199
reformation 53, 61, 126, 127, 140, 152
Reformatory Act (1858) 144
reformers 9, 29, 30, 33, 54, 55, 90, 135, 136, 172, 175
reform movement 3, 9
reform work 125, 144, 145, 148, 149, 151, 152, 155, 169
refuge 78, 95, 115, 116, 127, 133, 136, 137, 143, 156, 184
registered districts 124
regulations 2, 3, 23, 31, 33, 35, 44, 57, 58, 59, 63, 64, 65, 74, 75, 78, 79, 81, 86, 92, 93, 94, 95, 96, 97, 102, 103, 106, 109, 110, 113, 115, 118, 120, 122, 123, 124, 133, 134, 139, 143, 161, 176, 179, 184, 198
regulationists 121, 122, 176
religiosity 128
remedies 48, 50, 51, 54, 83, 113
repeal 117, 122, 123, 124, 151, 159, 164, 186, 188
Repeal Campaign 115, 118, 120, 162, 176, 178, 184, 196
repealers 120, 121, 122
repeal movement 117, 121, 123
repentance 92, 125, 128, 129, 130, 143, 148, 149, 151
reproduction 168, 186, 194
rescue 10, 127, 129, 151, 151, 175, 188, 197
Rescue Home 23, 152, 188, 189, 192
rescue work 2, 3, 10, 61, 81, 90, 92, 116, 119, 132, 163, 167, 181
resistance 71, 80, 117, 136, 155, 157, 184, 198, 199
respectability 3, 26, 62, 74, 130, 132, 143, 144, 157, 174, 175, 184, 186

respectable 26, 32, 34, 35, 58, 130, 135, 139, 145, 147, 153, 160, 165, 172, 186
respectable society 11
Ritchie, John 53, 54
Royal College of Physicians 5, 6
Royal College of Surgeons 5, 6, 187

salivation 13, 48, 51, 54
salivation wards 13, 51
salvarsan 52, 187, 198
salvation 22, 61, 92, 126, 127, 130, 140, 145
Salvation Army 182
sarsaparilla 47, 49, 50, 187
Scott, Thomas 22, 125
secretary 62, 63, 70, 78, 192
seduced 29, 142
seduction 28, 29, 33, 43, 81, 89, 90, 121, 175, 176, 177, 179, 180, 181
segregation 13, 62, 71, 124, 169
self-abuse 83, 168, 186
self-sacrifice 26, 151
separate spheres 126
sermon 20, 61, 78, 146, 192
sex abusers 174
sexes 25, 27, 28, 74, 83, 85, 87, 93, 122, 168, 185, 194, 195, 197
sexology 193, 194, 196
sexual 57, 93, 142, 159, 166, 167, 168, 171, 172, 173, 174, 175, 179, 184, 186, 193, 195, 196, 197, 199
sexual abuse 144, 167, 171, 172, 185
sexual activity 33, 42
sexual assault 174, 182
sexual behavior 58, 82, 155, 164, 194
sexual depravity 92
sexual desire 46, 82, 97
sexual deviance 173
sexual excess 82
sexual experience 33, 167
sexual exploitation 27, 102, 172, 179, 180, 181, 198

sexual feeling 31
sexual identity 82
sexual immorality 82
sexual initiation 88
sexual instinct 30, 82, 93, 195
sexual intercourse 35, 36, 38, 41, 48, 89, 147, 176, 182, 186
sexual labour *see* prostitution
sexual laxity 40
sexuality 24, 27, 58, 81, 102, 136, 143, 144, 159, 164, 168, 172, 176, 181, 182, 193, 194, 196, 199
sexually transmitted diseases 36, 57, 93, 97, 187
sexual misconduct 46, 99, 141, 155
sexual needs 10
sexual offenders 10
sexual promiscuity 9, 14, 23
sexual prudery 83
sexual relations 34
sexual transgression 14
sewing 144
Shield, The 120
silence 133, 144, 156
simple method 51
sinful 48, 136, 163
single moral standard 193, 195
single mothers 13
sinners 17, 57, 58, 61, 110, 132, 147, 149, 157
sins 9, 36, 58, 61, 140, 146, 148, 163
slavery 179
slave trade 178, 179
slave traffic 180
social evil 44
social reform 2, 119
Society of Apothecaries 5
Society for the Prevention of Cruelty to Children 183
Society for the Promotion of Christian Knowledge 9, 12, 15, 125

Index

Societies for the Promotion of Manners 9, 15, 125–126
Society for the Suppression of Vice (1802) 10, 183
sodomy 182, 193, 194
solicitation 35, 36, 122, 184, 196
"sore leg" 37
specialisation 3, 5, 6, 7, 92
specialist doctors 6
specialist hospitals 3, 5, 6, 8, 13, 14, 17
speculum 42, 87, 113
spermatorrhoea 83
Stansfeld, James 116, 123, 159
Stead, W.T. 88, 180, 181
stereotypes 25, 26, 29, 57
sterility 37 *see also* infertility
stigma 190
stigmatization 184
submissiveness 10, 74, 136, 151, 167
subordination 25, 26, 130, 137
subscribers 7, 22, 23, 59, 62, 64, 72, 125, 161
subscriptions 14, 15, 16, 60, 108, 152, 188, 192
subjected districts 111, 112, 121
Superintendent 41, 65, 66, 69, 71
surgeons 4, 8, 13, 16, 51, 53, 59, 60, 64, 66, 67, 73, 85, 86, 87, 99, 107, 109, 111, 112, 113, 187, 189
surveillance 8, 9, 57, 58, 79, 93, 94, 102, 114, 172, 173, 181, 186, 199; surveillants 145
suspension 123, 124
syphilis 36, 38, 39, 40, 41, 45, 47, 48, 49, 51, 57, 84, 87, 97, 112, 115, 121, 123, 151, 155, 173, 175, 176, 187, 190; congenital syphilis 36, 45, 46; hereditary syphilis 40, 45; neuro-syphilis 37; primary syphilis 36, 51, 67, 161 secondary syphilis 37, 41, 54, 67, 87, 161, 187; tertiary syphilis 37, 41, 45, 54, 87, 187; *see also* parasyphilitic disease; syphilitic chancre
syphilitic 41, 45, 46, 49, 50
syphilitic chancres *see* chancres

tabes dorsalis 45, 49, 187
Tait, William 29, 30, 89, 175
temperance 30, 90, 117, 170, 195
Temperance Movement 170, 184
texts of culture 39, 114, 130
Towns Police Clauses Act (1847) 35, 47
trade 88, 175, 178
traffic 118, 175, 178, 182
transgression 14, 28, 71, 74, 129, 197
treatments 1, 2, 3, 7, 8, 11. 13, 16, 17, 19, 37, 38, 41, 47, 48, 50, 51, 52, 54, 55, 66, 67, 69, 71, 72, 74, 76, 99, 100, 106, 111, 113, 114, 121, 123, 124, 127, 161, 186, 187, 189, 191, 197, 198

undeserving poor, the 10, 20, 40, 75, 184, 190, 199
uniforms 133, 143, 144
unity theory 40, 41
unrespectable 58

Vagrancy Act (1824) 27, 35
Vagrancy Law Amendment Act (1898) 196
venereal care 24
venereal disease 1, 2, 3, 6, 11, 12, 13, 14, 16, 17, 19, 33, 36, 39, 40, 41, 43, 44, 45, 46, 47, 48, 49, 50, 51, 52, 53, 54, 55, 58, 66, 74, 78, 80, 89, 93, 94, 96, 97, 100, 102, 103, 106, 107, 109, 110, 112, 113, 115, 117, 120, 121, 129, 132, 134, 149, 150, 155, 160, 173, 174, 175, 176, 179, 187, 190, 197, 198, 199; patients 11, 14, 16, 17, 18, 72, 84
venereal facilities 17, 70, 91, 113

venereal hospital 128
venereal legislation 92–93, 96, 108
venereal poison 42, 47, 93
venereal wards 11, 20, 24
venereal warts 36, 38, 87
venereology 97, 109, 187, 194
vices 9, 18, 28, 58, 90, 109, 119, 129, 150, 186, 195
victims 28, 29, 36, 39, 46, 61, 89, 93, 110, 120, 130, 144, 147, 172, 174, 176, 179, 180, 181
violence 27, 34, 93, 137, 174
violation 120, 173, 180
virgins 29
virtue 26, 86, 151
Voluntary Hospital Movement 7
voluntary hospitals 3, 6, 8, 14, 15, 17, 18, 20, 24, 68, 73, 191, 193
voluntary subscriptions 7, 13

wages of sin 34
War Office 24, 103, 106, 107, 108, 149, 152
wards 5, 13, 14, 15, 16, 21, 23, 24, 60, 61, 62, 63, 67, 68, 69, 71, 73, 79, 99, 101, 108, 128, 142, 149, 162
Wesley, John 19
white slavery 3, 88, 171, 179, 180, 181, 196
white slaves 175
white slave trade 179, 180
Wilde, Oscar 195, 196
Wolstenholme, Elizabeth 116, 117, 185
Women's Protest 118, 120
women's sphere 70
workhouse infirmaries 12, 13, 52, 101, 102
Workhouse Test Act 12, 78, 99, 102, 116
workhouses 8, 11, 12, 13, 14, 33, 58, 64, 72, 91, 100, 101, 102, 134, 145, 150, 155, 165, 166, 187

www.ingramcontent.com/pod-product-compliance
Ingram Content Group UK Ltd.
Pitfield, Milton Keynes, MK11 3LW, UK
UKHW021845140426
5217IPUK00022B/1595